An Assessment of Services Provided to Children Affected and Infected by HIV/AIDS in Windhoek, Namibia

Cynthy Haihambo
University of Namibia

Jacqueline Hayden
University of Western Sydney

Barnabas Otaala
University of Namibia

Roderick Zimba
University of Namibia

Published by

University of Namibia Press

Private Bag 13301
Pioneerspark
Windhoek, Namibia

Supported by

WORLD FORUM
FOUNDATION

World Forum

University of Namibia

University of
Western Sydney
Bringing knowledge to life

Centre for Social Justice and Social Change, University of Western Sydney

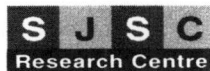

S J S C
Research Centre

ISBN: 99916 – 67 – 05 - 9

First Published in 2004

Published by
University of Namibia Press
Private Bag 13301
Pioneerspark
Windhoek, Namibia

Printed by
John Meinert Printing (1999)
Windhoek, Namibia

Graphics Assistant
John Rittmann

ISBN 99916 - 67 - 05 - 9

Photographs in the front and back covers by Jacqueline Hayden

TABLE OF CONTENTS

ACRONYMS / ABBREVIATIONS

AIDS	Acquired Immune Deficiency Syndrome
CAFO	The Church Alliance for Orphans
DRC	Democratic Republic of the Congo
ECDNA	Early Childhood Development Network for Africa
EFA	Education For All
HIV	Human Immunodeficiency Syndrome
IEC	Information Education and Communication
MHSS	Ministry of Health and Social Services
MINEDAF	Ministers of Education in Africa
NGOs	Non-Governmental Organizations
OVCs	Orphans and Other Vulnerable Children
RA	Research Assistant
rh	residential houses
sh	safe houses
UCRC	United Nations Convention on the Rights of Children
UNAIDS	United Nations Joint Programme on HIV/AIDS
UNESCO	United Nations Educational, Scientific and Cultural Organization
UNICEF	United Nations Children's Educational Fund
USAID	United States Agency for International Development
UWS	University of Western Sydney

ACKNOWLEDGEMENTS

The authors would like to acknowledge the contributions of various institutions that contributed to the success of the pilot project which resulted in the publication of this book.

We express our appreciation to the World Forum Foundation on Early Care and Education, which provided funds under the World Forum Networking Project to which we applied for financial support. The Networking Fund is sponsored by Pademelon Press and supported by the New South Wales Department of Community Services, to both of whom we express our thanks.

The University of Namibia as part of its contribution to the project, provided accommodation and office space to one of the authors (Dr Hayden) during the field phase of the project when she came to the University as Visiting Professor. We express our deep appreciation for this generous support. The Social Justice and Social Change Research Centre, University of Western Sydney, Australia, agreed to fund the publication of the report. We are deeply indebted to them for this support.

Various individuals, either singly or collectively also contributed to the success of the project, and we would like to acknowledge them. These include, the Research Assistants - Joyce Tseitseimou; Belinda Kandundu; and Christine Neufeld. Professor Jan Mason, Mr Robert Urquhart, Mr Jason White and Dr Katey De Gidia from the Social Justice and Social Change Research Centre, University of Western Sydney, Australia, are thanked for their assistance and generous support. We thank Aline Amutenya and John Rittmann of the University of Namibia for getting the report ready for publication.

Finally, the authors wish to acknowledge the support and assistance of all participants in this study who contributed time and valuable information at every stage. Special thanks go to the twelve children whose openness and honesty added immensely to the findings of this study and whose sharing of their vision for a better future was an inspiration to us all.

Cynthy Haihambo
University of Namibia
Windhoek

Jacqueline Hayden
University of Western
Sydney, Australia

Barnabas Otaala
University of Namibia
Windhoek

Roderick F Zimba
University of Namibia
Windhoek

ABOUT THE AUTHORS

Ms Cynthy Kaliinasho Haihambo was born and raised in Windhoek, Namibia. After completion of her school career, she went to the then Khomasdal Teachers Training College, and then proceeded to do a Bachelor of Education (Hons.) degree at the University of Namibia. She served as a secondary school teacher just before and after the attainment of Namibia's independence. She then went to the University of Oslo in Norway, where she completed a Master's degree in Philosophy of Special Needs Education in 1996.

Currently she is a Lecturer and Researcher in the Department of Educational Psychology and Special Needs Education. As upcoming teacher trainer and researcher, she has conducted research in various areas of Special Needs Education, HIV/AIDS, Street Children, the Girl Child and Orphans and other vulnerable children. She believes strongly in the development of intervention programmes for young children and youth at risk or in need of care.

Dr Jacqueline Hayden is Associate Professor in Child and Youth Studies at the University of Western Sydney (UWS) and has researched or worked in program delivery in several nations including Australia, Canada, New Zealand, Mauritius, South Africa, West Indies, Zimbabwe and the Rwandan refugee camps in the DRC. Jacqueline is a founding member of the Social Justice and Social Change Research Centre and the Director of the Healthy Childhood Research Group at UWS

(www.healthychildhood.org). Her most recent book is **Landscapes in Early Childhood Education** (Peter Lang). In 2004 she was a visiting Professor at University of Namibia.

Professor Barnabas Otaala trained in Kampala, London, and New York, and divides his work today between Africa and England, and America.

During a 30-year plus career in Early Childhood Care and Development, Professor Otaala has concentrated on the African continent but has also advised at an international level. He has been especially involved as an international adviser in the use of the child-to-child approach developed by the Child-to-Child Trust at the Institute of Education, University of London.

Professor Otaala holds a B.A. (London) degree and a Dip.Ed. (East Africa) from Makerere University, Kampala,Uganda. He also holds an M.A. (Developmental Psychology) and Ed.D. (Educational Psychology) from Teachers College, Columbia University in the City of New York (USA).

He was Professor of Educational Psychology and Special Education, Faculty of Education, University of Namibia until the end of December, 1998. In 1995 – 1998, he was also the Dean of Education, University of Namibia.

Professor Otaala has previously worked at Makerere University, Kampala, Uganda; University of Botswana, Gaborone, Botswana; and the National Teachers Training College, Maseru, Lesotho.

He is currently Coordinator of the Unit for Improving Teaching and Learning at the University of Namibia as well as the Chairperson of the University's HIV/AIDS Task Force.

Roderick Futula Zimba is a Professor of Educational Psychology and Director of Postgraduate Studies at the University of Namibia. He has, over the years, taught undergraduate and postgraduate courses in Educational Psychology, Educational Social Psychology, Educational Research Methodology, Early Childhood Development and Special Needs Education. Professor Zimba has considerable experience in conducting research on childcare and development, special needs education, inclusive education, the impact of HIV/AIDS on youth in school, the education of orphans and other vulnerable children, discipline in schools and values education. Furthermore Professor Zimba has participated and continues to participate in community service activities pertaining to education reforms in Namibia, educationally marginalized children and the Examinations Board of Namibia.

FOREWORD

Three years ago ten members of the Early Childhood Development Network for Africa (ECDNA) met in Johannesburg, South Africa, to launch this initiative which contributes towards identification of current levels of support and intervention in favour of orphans and vulnerable children in six countries in Sub-Saharan Africa (Uganda, Kenya, Namibia, South Africa, Swaziland, and Mauritius).

The initiative provides the network with an opportunity of developing methodologies to initiate, carry out, and evaluate a series of linked action research projects for children affected by HIV/AIDS, and their carers. Information thus collected would provide a database and could be used for advocacy, training of staff, and development of policies in several sectors such as Information, Education and Communication (IEC); Education For All (EFA); Nutrition, Health and Youth programs.

Since the first meeting members have contributed to various events, forums, and workshops. These include meetings at the Hague, Netherlands, in December 2001; UNESCO, in Paris, France, May 2002; the second International Early Childhood Conference in Africa, Eritrea in October 2002; the Conference of Ministers of Education in Africa (MINEDAF VIII), Dar es Salaam, in December 2002, and the World Forum on Early Care and Education in Acapulco, Mexico, April, 2003. It was at this latter Forum that Jacqueline Hayden from Australia and Barnabas Otaala from Namibia submitted a proposal to the World Forum Networking Fund. The submission was based on the Namibia proposal which had been approved by the Early Childhood Development Network for Africa (ECDNA) meeting in UNESCO, Paris in May 2002.

The Networking Fund of the World Forum on Early Care and Education furthers the mission of the World Forum to foster an ongoing global exchange of ideas by supporting international networking projects. The Networking Fund is sponsored by Pademelon Press and supported by the New South Wales Department of Community Services, Australia.

The proposal for the project entitled "*An Assessment of Services Offered to Children (0- 8) Affected and Infected by HIV/AIDS in Namibia*" was the successful recipient of the Networking Fund grant for 2003. The project was further supported by the University of Western Sydney, Social Justice and Social Change Research Centre and by the University of Namibia. Barnabas Otaala and Jacqueline Hayden were joined by Cynthy Haihambo and Roderick Zimba to form the research team for this project.

From the work that emerged from our project the title for this book could have been: "*Young Children and HIV/AIDS: A Case Study of the Experiences of Children aged 0-8 years Who are Infected or Affected by HIV/AIDS in Windhoek, Namibia*".

The reason for this is that the results present information which goes beyond an assessment of services in Windhoek. The study actually achieves a number of goals:

1.   It presents an argument about the importance of research which focuses on the 0 – 8 year old age group;

2.   It argues for the value of taking an ecological approach to data gathering for this age group;

3.   It provides (tested) strategies for gathering data on this age group and about sensitive issues;

4.   It provides a typography (adapted from a number of sources especially for this study) which serves as a framework for an assessment of services and other influences upon the health and well being of young children and their caregivers;

5.   It incorporates voices of the children and their caregivers – and includes narratives which provide a picture of what it is like to be an orphaned and vulnerable child (OVC) or to be a caregiver of an OVC under a number of diverse situations;

6.   It analyses the experiences of the children and the caregivers against the typography of human rights and needs;

7.   It differentiates experiences of the target population according to diverse living situations and provides analyses and recommendations for these diverse settings and situations; and

8.   Lastly, it provides an assessment of current services delivery to the target population and makes recommendations to facilitate a targeted approach to meeting the needs and rights of the target population;

We, however, decided to keep the original title reflected in this book. This is because, among others things, it tallies with the larger proposed original study, for which we are still seeking funding.

In undertaking the project reported here we believed there would be a direct outcome for children aged (0 – 8) affected and infected by HIV/AIDS. We also envision that the processes and the information, which are "trialled" by this project, will have long-term sustainable outcomes. We are now in the process of using the findings to seek additional funds for extended studies of this nature. The study can be replicated in other parts and regions of Namibia, and indeed in other parts of southern Africa where the HIV/AIDS pandemic is rampant.

                                                                                    Barnabas Otaala

INTRODUCTION

A number of studies have been published about the plight of children infected and affected by HIV/AIDS. These studies have been helpful in providing information on incidence and prevalence, identifying the complex and interacting outcomes for children, highlighting issues for attention and support and articulating the implications for social/economic development on a local and often national level (see Reference list).

It is now well known that HIV/AIDS has grave implications for children beyond infection. Huge numbers have been orphaned and/or have been subject to trauma, disruption of lifestyle, poverty, stigmatisation, abuse and other forms of victimisation.

During the time period that the devastating effects of the HIV/AIDS pandemic on children worldwide, and especially in sub-Sahara Africa, was becoming known, a surge of research into early childhood development was gaining global recognition.

During the early 1980s brain imaging techniques confirmed that experiences during the earliest years of life influence permanent neurological functioning. It became clear that many biomedical, psychosocial, emotional and intellectual outcomes in adolescence and adulthood can be traced back to the early childhood experiences of individuals.

Oddly, conclusions about the importance and long-term effects of the early years have not been correlated to research concerning implications of the HIV/AIDS pandemic on young children[1].

This study presents a first step in attempting to corroborate what has been called "the most significant issue facing children today" (USAID, UNAIDS& UNICEF, 2002) with our current knowledge about the outcome of experiences during early life.

Using open-ended questions, which facilitated the articulation of narratives or stories from children and their caretakers, the study provides an insight into what it means to be young, orphaned, infected or affected in other ways by HIV/AIDS. Situations and settings are described and conclusions are drawn about the ways by which global principles of healthy environments and quality settings for children are being and can be met under current conditions.

Underlying assumptions

The study rides on some basic assumptions. Children who are diagnosed as HIV positive are seen nonetheless to have the potential to live fulfilling and even long lives. There is no rationale for compromising the quality of their day-to-day experiences which have both current andfuture outcomes.

The second assumption is that despite many common issues for orphaned and vulnerable children

---

[1] A recent publication is a notable exception to this gap in the literature. See Consultative Group on Early Childhood Development (2002) *Coordinators Notebook on HIV/AIDS and Early Childhood Vol 26*

(OVC) as recorded in numerous studies, each child's situation (and needs) are seen to be unique to that child. The study does not attempt to uncover any overriding solution, situation or program for the target group. Rather the study attempts to provide a snapshot of a variety of programs which are currently serving children and to suggest ways to maximise the current capacity of these situations.

This information, it is hoped, will provide ideas about processes for the development of further research and programs which target similar populations in diverse contexts.

REVIEW OF THE LITERATURE

Typography of human needs and rights

In 1970, Maslow articulated the hierarchy of human needs which culminates in the self-actualized personality (Maslow, 1970). The *UN Charter of Human Rights* (United Nations General Assembly, 1948) and the *UN Convention on the Rights of the Child* (United Nations General Assembly, 1989) have identified basic rights which reflect these needs. Human beings need and have a right to conditions that ensure survival – nourishment, shelter, protection from violence and harm. Beyond this they need conditions that allow for growth and development – adequate supplies of food and water, disease free environments and access to health services. Children need nurturance and protection from adults. All human beings need positive, reciprocal affiliation with others in order to develop and sustain emotional health and well being. Exposure to conditions conducive to cognitive development and stimulation (learning) and membership within a family and community grouping are basic needs at this level. As children mature they have a right to free and compulsory formal education. They need to be exposed to positive role models and to engage in activities which provide skills for living. Human beings need to be able to test and develop their unique talents and individual characteristics. Finally human beings need and have a right to seek conditions that allows them to fulfill their potential and follow their own interests. To do this they need to have freedom of expression, choice and movement. At all stages, the individual's right to participate in decisions affecting his or her life need to be honoured.

This typography of human needs and rights is illustrated in Box 1 (adapted from (Maslow, 1970; United Nations General Assembly, 1948, 1989).

Box 1: Typography of human rights and needs.

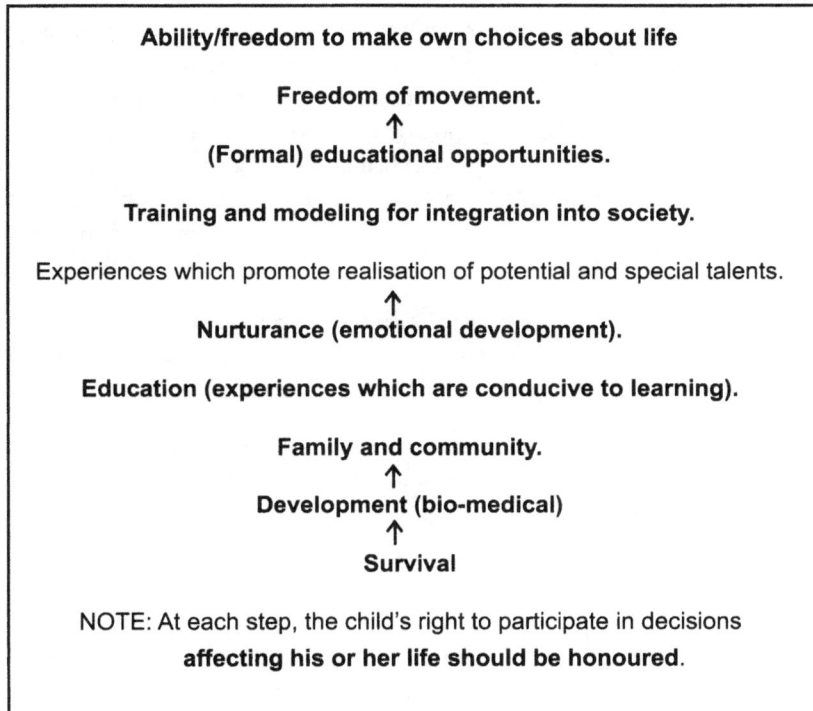

Ability/freedom to make own choices about life

Freedom of movement.
↑
(Formal) educational opportunities.

Training and modeling for integration into society.

Experiences which promote realisation of potential and special talents.
↑
Nurturance (emotional development).

Education (experiences which are conducive to learning).

Family and community.
↑
Development (bio-medical)
↑
Survival

NOTE: At each step, the child's right to participate in decisions **affecting his or her life should be honoured**.

HIV/AIDS and young children

The statistics on HIV/AIDS and its impact on children have been documented for many years. Of an estimated 40 million people worldwide living with HIV today, more than four million are children under the age of 15.   More than 13 million children under the age of 15 have lost one or both parents to AIDS, most of them in sub-Saharan Africa.

The *State of the World's Children* (United Nations International Children's Fund, 2002) continues to name HIV/AIDS as the most critical issue facing children today. The figures of affected and infected children continue to rise. By 2010, it is estimated that more than 25 million children will be orphaned as a result of the pandemic. With infection rates rising, HIV/AIDS will continue to cause suffering among children.

The impacts of AIDS on children are complex and multifaceted. The intensity of the impacts is correlated to poverty, loss of social/cultural traditions, stigmatisation and other issues which are particular to each situation.

There is ample evidence that children affected and infected by HIV/AIDS are often denied   basic rights. These include an inherent right to life, to experiences for optimal development and to an enriching standard of living and protection from various forms of harm, abuse, neglect, exploitation and deprivation (United Nations General Assembly, 1989).

Infected and affected children suffer psychosocial distress and are at risk of exclusion, abuse, discrimination, and stigmatisation. As parents and other family members become ill, children take on greater responsibility for income generation, food production and care of family members, loss of adequate nutrition, basic health care, housing and clothing, the risk of being denied an education, loss of inheritance, abuse and/or the effects of running a child-headed household are some of the impacts of the pandemic on young children (USAID, UNAIDS, & UNICEF, 2002). Ironically, some services which target these children have exacerbated their exposure to abuse, neglect and exploitation (The Children's Institute, 2001)

A South African study reported that the psychological impact on a child of losing a parent to HIV/AIDS often goes unacknowledged. Children were shown to be discriminated against at home, in schools, shops, taxis and other settings. This stigmatisation borders on abuse.

It has been shown that children aged 5-14 years who have lost one or both parents are less likely to be in school and more likely to be working 40 hours or more per week.

A survey of 646 orphaned and 1,239 non-orphaned children in Kenya found that 52 percent of orphaned children were not in school, while only 2 percent of non-orphaned children were not enrolled. (Lust, Huffman and O'Gara, 2000)

Affected children who do attend school have high rates of absenteeism because of sickness at home or because they are sick themselves. When they do attend classes they may have trouble concentrating because of distress and worries or because of alienation from their peers. Teachers who are uninformed of their home circumstances are likely to punish children for lack of attention, falling asleep in class or not completing homework (Summary of the National Children's Forum on HIV/AIDS, 2001).

It has been shown that children who move into relative or other 'foster care' situations can suffer from stigmatisation and discrimination in food allocation, education and workload in comparison with the foster parents' own children. (Subbarao, Mattimore and Plangemann, 2001)

Other studies have shown that affected children who disclose their situation in order to seek support (such as with school fees) are often subject to further abuse and discrimination.

Misconceptions about the spread of HIV/AIDS add to discrimination against children who are often shunned by other children and/or refused entry to schools and kindergartens. Infection or association with HIV can be viewed as a punishment 'from God' or a result of being bewitched.

While the research on the effects of HIV/AIDS for 0 to 5 year olds is scarce, some statistics have been gathered on outcomes believed to be associated with the pandemic. These include morbidity, stunting, nutritional wasting, and failure to thrive (See Lusk & O'Gara, 2002). That children in the earliest years of life are especially vulnerable to the effects of the HIV/AIDS pandemic has not been highlighted in most studies. This seems surprising in light of the current knowledge base about the long-term effects on the early years of life.

The early years of life

Brain imaging techniques have confirmed that the earliest years of life are a critical stage in the determination of biological, neurological, psychological and emotional/social health and well-being for individuals and that key environmental factors and nurturing experiences during early years are significantly correlated to psychological and biomedical outcomes in later life. Early experiences including bonding and attachment, the development of security and trust through consistent care taking, freedom to interact with surroundings, predicability, success experiences, responsiveness, exposure to opportunities for cognitive and emotional development and other nurturing interactions are now known to be significantly related to long term developmental outcomes (Love, Schochet, & Meckstroth, 1996; Marmot & Wilkinson, 1999; Pence, 1999; Shonkoff & Phillips, 2000; Wadsworth, 1999; Zigler & Gilman, 1998).

The early years can form a protective base for lifelong stress and trauma. Children who have had stable, nurturing care in early life show more resilience to traumatic events which occur in subsequent years (Barry, 1996; Carnegie Corporation of New York, 2000; McCain & Mustard, 1999; Schweinhart & Weikart, 1993; UNICEF, 1994).

The importance of social connections

Similarly, studies have highlighted the long-term outcomes associated with connectedness of families and individuals. Young children whose caregivers are accepted as members of a close knit group or community have been shown to be less likely to become socially alienated and/or depressed in later life (Leeder, 1998; Parcel & Menaghan, 1994; Wong, 1998).

Recent research in western settings has identified the correlation between social connections and the health and well-being of individuals. Social capital, or the store of goodwill and co-operation between people, is seen an enabler for fostering the emotional and practical resources that support effective functioning in day-to-day life. This in turn contributes to strong, active, 'healthy' communities (Cox, 1995; Wilkinson, 2000). Living in a healthy, connected community is co related to psychosocial, emotional, behavioural and biomedical outcomes in children and families (Vinson, 1999; Wilkinson, 2000). Social connections, including access to close friends, nuclear and extended family, co-workers, clubs, church, and regular supportive interactions with other people, have been reported to influence the life expectancy of individuals. Conversely, social isolation and/or a lack of social capital have been shown to be related to the development of poor mental health and increased rates of morbidity and mortality (Marmot & Wilkinson, 1999; Maton, 2000; Nicholson, Tually, & Vimpani, 2000; Wilkinson, 2000). In a recent US study individuals who lack social connections were shown to have two to three times the risk of dying from all causes compared with well-connected individuals (Kawachi, Kennedy, & Glass, 1999).

Access to health promoting settings

In most minority (Western) world countries, the majority of children under the age of 6 years have access to programs offered through early childhood services. These programs tend to include trained caregivers whose role is to provide nurturance and stimulation to small groups of children, often in purpose built establishments. For the most part these services are regulated and monitored by government authorities and comply with national or regional standards which relate to health and safety but also to minimum space per child requirements, adult-to-child ratios, training requirements for staff (in many cases) and equipment and programming (in most areas) (Hayden & Macdonald, 2001; Hayden & Macdonald, 2000).

Global indicators of quality care for children in group settings

In the resource rich nations where childcare tends to be formal and institutionalised, indicators of 'quality care' for early childhood services have been assessed over several decades. Indicators have focused on 'micro' items within the 'physical environment'; the quality of the air and light, floor space per child, equipment and safety issues; consistent caregiving, adult-to-child ratios, training levels of staff, industrial issues which support teamwork and decrease staff turnover, level of child-directed versus teacher-directed activities, balance of attention to all developmental areas (social, emotional physical, creative, cognitive and spiritual), attention to hygiene, nutrition, and health needs of the child.

When contextual relevance is recognised, early childhood services in less resource-rich environments, such as those in developing countries, can still rate highly on 'micro' characteristics of high quality. The key is to measure the service against community norms of safety and hygiene. An understanding of early childhood development issues and genuine interest in providing good care is another indicator for services in resource- poor circumstances (see Hayden, 2002).

In the past few decades meta- analyses of outcomes and longitudinal studies have revealed that quality service extends beyond classroom 'micro' practices and incorporate 'macro' items which are family and community oriented:

Early childhood service delivery is now known to be associated with the facilitation of environments that enhance social capital, prevent social alienation and increase opportunities for inclusion and the development of networks and support for families of young children.

Thus early childhood services that produce sustained benefits for children and families are those which provide support to parents and caretakers, build trust relationships for all involved and facilitate community linkages for families with young children. The activities for achieving these differ radically between settings (especially between those in developed and those in developing nations), but the underlying principles remain. Quality experiences for groups of young children which focus on communication, collaboration and participation with families and with related health and community service providers are now considered to be a positive and supportive component of healthy environments for very young children (Clarke & Campbell, 1989; Dahlberg, Moss, & Pence, 1999; Doherty-

Derkowski, 1995; Ferguson, Horwood, & Lynskey, 1994; Hayden & Macdonald, 2001; Lero, 2000; McBride, 1999; Moss, 1995; Parcel & Menaghan, 1994; Pence, 1999; Shonkoff & Phillips, 2000; Wong & Patterson, 2000).

The following principles are associated with quality group care in both developed and developing nations (World Bank, 2000,adapted by Hayden, 2002).

These principles are seen to allow for contextual relevance within diverse situations and to be independent of resource allocations. While the principles generally apply to non-residential programs, there is no reason to discount their relevance to "live-in" situations for orphans and vulnerable children.

Early childhood programs with the following characteristics are most likely to be health promoting for children and families when:

1.   *Programs are community driven and highly participatory*

       Programs are effective when communities and/or caregivers retain ownership of the program. In some cases this includes physically building the premises, recruiting the (local) teacher, organising training and ensuring upkeep of the setting and environment. This intensive inter action with the program develops commitment from the users and has been shown to contrib ute to success and sustainability.

2.   *Programs emphasise a wide diversity of areas concerning children's health and well-being*

       Early childhood health promoting programs need to include services which meet a wide diver sity of local and regional needs. Family reunification, foster care services, child and maternal health care, nutritional and dental programs, income-generating schemes, building support networks for parents, and many other activities, can fall under the umbrella of early childhood programs.

3.   *Programs emphasise strategic communications for awareness-raising*

       Effective programs include a communication, awareness-raising component through the dis semination of information about healthy practices for children and families. Community meet ings, and information sharing workshops should be part of the program. On a wider scale,early childhood programs can make use of radio, posters, television, cartoons and/or print, video and information technology to promote child-centred messages. Popular drama and street theatre have been successful in disseminating health-promoting messages in areas where mass communication is not part of daily life.

4.   *Programs have links to community programs including schools*

Effective early childhood programs are linked to health and nutrition services and to schools. These links have been successful in increasing school attendance rates and in decreasing morbidity in young children.

5.   *Programs provide training opportunities for sustainability*

Effective early childhood programs have a system for sustainability and perpetuation. They rely upon a number of workers at all levels and, to the extent possible, upon multiple sources of funding and support. The inclusion of trainees and apprentices ensures that programs can continue beyond the availability of any one individual and/or that enhanced or increased pro grams can be implemented when new needs or new clients emerge. (See Box 2)

Box 2: Characteristics of effective early childhood programs

---

1. **Programs are community driven and highly participatory.**

2. **Programs emphasise a wide diversity of areas concerning children's health and well-being**

3. **Programs emphasise strategic communications for awareness raising**

4. **Programs have links to community programs including schools.**

5. **Programs provide training opportunities for sustainability.**

(World Bank, 2000, adapted by Hayden, 2002)

The situation in Namibia

The tables below show recent statistics recorded for Namibia. Notably, the life expectancy in Namibia has decreased by an astonishing three years since 1970. This is believed to be directly related to the increased incidence of HIV/AIDS. The number of children affected because of high mortality rates of adults will have risen accordingly.

Similarly there is reason to believe that the statistics on incidence and prevalence of HIV/AIDS and related numbers of orphans could be substantially higher than records show. This is because of the stigma attached to the disease and the concomitant reluctance to test and/or to disclose.

(*from UNICEF, *The State of the World's Children 2003*, pgs 86, 102, 112)

Table 1: Basic indicators for Namibia

Under-5 mortality rank	Under-5 mortality rate		Infant mortality rate (under 1)		Total population (thousands) 2001	Annual no. of births (thousands) 2001	Annual no. of under-5 deaths (thousands) 2001	GNI per capita (US$) 2001	Life expectancy at birth (years) 2001	Total adult literacy rate 2000	Net primary school enrolment/ attendance (%) 1995-2001*
	1960	2001	1960	2001							
69	206	67	129	55	1788	63	4	1960	45	82	80

Table 2: Demographic Indicators for Namibia

Under-5 mortality rank	Population (thousands) 2001		Population annual growth rate (%)		Crude death rate		Crude birth rate		Life expectancy		Total fertility rate 2001	% of population on urbanised 2001	Average annual growth rate of urban population %	
	Under 18	Under 5	1970-90	1990-2001	1970	2001	1970	2001	1970	2001			1970-90	1990-2001
69	900	282	2.8	2.4	18	18	44	35	48	45	5.0	31	4.6	3.9

Table 3: Incidence and prevalence of HIV/Aids in Namibia

Adult prevalence rate (15-19 years), end-2001	Estimated no. of people living with HIV/AIDS, end 2001		HIV prevalence among pregnant women (aged 15-24), major urban areas			ORPHANS	
	Adults and children (0-49 years)	Children (0-14 years)	Year (no. of sites surveyed)	Median 15-19 years)	Median (20-24 years)	Children orphaned by AIDS (0-14 years) 2001	Orphan school attendance rate as a % of non-orphan attendance rate (1995-2001*)
22.5	230 000	30 000	2000(n)	11.9	20.3	47 000	Not recorded

Information specific to children in Namibia has been documented in a variety of ways.

Recently the Ministry of Health and Social Services developed a Five-Year Strategic Plan (2001-2006) for orphans and vulnerable children (OVCs). This contains program proposals covering 2002-2003 and plans for monitoring and evaluating the quality of service provision. (Ministry of Health and Social Services, 2001)

A comprehensive directory of resources for Namibian OVCs has been published for several years (See Steinitz, 1998; Kandtu, 2000) The most recent publication identifies the services provided by Catholic AIDS Action and other Non-Government Organisations (NGOs). Over nine thousand (9885) children and 1625 family units were registered at time of publication (Steinitz, 2002)

Anecdotal evidence shows a growing commitment by organisations and caregivers to address the needs of young OVCs, especially those infected and affected by HIV/AIDS. However, from the information available, it is not clear whether or how services are differentiated for the youngest (0- 8 years) population, nor which, if any, resources specifically target this age group. Nor could information on the quality of resources available to OVCs be located. Information about situations and services for children before they enter the school system is particularly difficult to access.[2] Qualitative data that includes descriptions of the experiences of caregivers and/or narratives that incorporate children's perspectives could not be found.

This study was developed to address this gap in the literature. An ecological framework was used to document the supports, constraints and experiences of service providers, caregivers and OVCs aged 0- 8 years old. The urban area of Khomas region (a designated high prevalence area for HIV/AIDS) was targeted for this preliminary study.[3]

RESEARCH FRAMEWORK

The study was developed as a pilot for a proposed larger project entitled *An Assessment of Services for Young Orphans, Older Orphans and other Children Affected and Infected by HIV/AIDS in the Caprivi, Erongo, Karas, Kavango, Khomas, Ohangwena, Omaheke and Oshana Regions of Namibia* (Zimba, Otaala et al., 2002) (see Appendix II)

---

[2] Statistics which have been gathered on services and/or needs of OVCs in Namibia tend not to differentiate between particular age groups. One exception is the recent study on Namibia Child Activities (Ministry of Labour, 2000). The description of working conditions in this document includes categories for children aged 6-9 years. (see table XX on page).

[3] This study is serving as a pilot for addressing the research and support needs for this population on a national level. See Zimba, R., Otaala B, et al (2002) *An Assessment of Services for Young Orphans, Older Orphans and other Children Affected and Infected by HIV/AIDS in the Caprivi, Erongo, Karas, Kavango, Khomas, Ohangwena, Omaheke and Oshana Regions of Namibia* (Zimba, Otaala et al, 2002)

The pilot study differs from the original proposal in a few ways: It includes a discrete geographical area (urban sites in Khomas region); it targets children in the early years of life (0-8 years of age) and it focuses on qualitative data gathering methods.

In light of the literature which identifies the long-term effects of experiences in the earliest years of life, the pilot sought to assess what it is like to be young, orphaned and/or HIV possitive and what it s like to be a caregiver for such a child. As part of the data gathering, information about supporting agents and organisations was included in this investigation.

The ecological approach was deemed to provide an appropriate framework for this study (Bronfenbrenner, 1979; 1986). In an ecological framework analyses of children's' experiences go beyond individual measures to include investigation of the systems or environmental factors which have a direct and indirect impact upon the child.

Bronfenbrenner identified four levels or *systems which* constitute an ecological framework. These include the micro-, meso-, exo- and macro-systems. Each system and the interactions between the systems need to be taken into account when assessing the experiences of any child or group of children.

For the purposes of this study data was gathered on each system as follows:

1)   Micro-system: Information about the child;

2)   Meso- system: Information about the setting, including caregivers;

3)   Exo-system: Information about programs and services which directly affect the setting, caregiver and the child;

4)   Macro-system: Information about the larger context including, community attitudes, policy directions and strategies which influence service planning and delivery.

Research goals

As it was a pilot, the study had two sets of goals. The first set of goals relates to investigating experiences and issues for the target population (children aged 0-8 years in Khomas region) within an ecological framework. These goals reflect those of the original proposal[4], with some adaptation: They include

1. To identify services and programs for young orphans and other children infected and affected by HIV/AIDS in the selected region:

    -   to assess current funding issues associated with such services and programs.

2. To describe the experience of being a young orphan or other child infected and affected by HIV/AIDS in the selected region:

    -   to assess how services provided to these children take into account the rights and needs of the children under current conditions.

3. To describe the experience of being a caregiver for young orphans or other children infected and affected by HIV/AIDS in the selected region:

    -   to assess how the rights and needs of the caregivers are being met under current conditions.

4. To identify gaps or potential gaps in service provision to the target population and make recommendations for enhancing quality of life and services for these children.

---

[4] Goals of the original proposal are
1. To identify programs that provide services to young orphans aged 0-8 years, and other children infected and affected by HIV/AIDS throughout Namibia

2. To delineate the nature of services that are provided to the young orphans, older orphans and other children affected and infected by HIV/AIDS.

3. To identify the strengths and constraints within households, communities, governmental and non governmental service providers in their ability to meet the needs for cognitive development, psychosocial development, and other well being needs of orphans and other children affected and infected by HIV/AIDS

4. To assess how services provided to young orphans, older orphans and other children affected and infected by HIV/AIDS take into account the rights of the children, especially the rights that pertain to protection from abuse, neglect, exploitation, stigmatisation and discrimination;

5. To propose policy and program strategies for serving Namibian children affected and infected by HIV/AIDS and generate information towards the development of a National policy on children. (See Appendix II)

A further goal for the pilot study was to identifi effective methods for data gathering which can be applied when the study expands as per the original proposal.(The expanded study will include affected and infected children up to the age of 18 years in several regions of Namibia.)

METHODOLOGY

Selection of participating organisations and respondents

Organisations were included through a snowball technique. The major organisations that deal with children in the region were contacted and asked to nominate other contacts (organisations and centres) which it might be appropriate to include in the study. These contacts were similarly asked to nominate others.

Every nominated contact was contacted by telephone or in person to establish if they met the criteria for inclusion in the study. Those deemed appropriate were invited to participate.

Participating organisations were asked to name settings where children aged 0-8 years who were infected or affected by HIV/AIDS could be found. The settings were approached by researchers and, where appropriate, organisation representatives. Those who met the criteria were invited to participate in the study.

Setting operators were asked to identify three caregivers and three children who would be eligible to participate (respondents). Setting operators spoke to the respondents to secure their permission for an interview. Children were not forewarned but were invited by the caregiver or the interviewers to take part on the day of the interview[5].

Participants and respondents included representatives or directors of large and small organisations,caregivers from three settings and children age 3 years to 9 years of age. In total 35

---

[5] All invited children participated eagerly. Some additional children asked if they could be interviewed as well. These interviews took place but the data was not included in the study.

interviews were conducted as shown in Table 4 below.

Table 4: Number of Participants/Respondents

Interviews conducted	Number interviewed
Representatives /Directors of organisations (large and small)	10
Caregivers - in non-community based settings - in safe houses - in residential houses Total	3 4 6 13
Children aged 3-9 years	12
TOTAL	**35**

Non-community based settings included orphanages and other public institutions. Caregivers are paid salaries and receive other benefits (such as accommodation for themselves and their families).

Safe houses are houses which belong to or are rented by caregivers who live on the premises and receive allowances on a per child basis for an allocated number of children. The situation is deemed to be temporary, until children can be placed with relatives and/or can be adopted or fostered.

Residential houses are indistinguishable from other houses in any community. They provide care for children who may be related to the resident of the house or have another connection. Caregivers in residential houses are generally not provided with formal means of support.

Criteria for participation

Organisations included in the study were those providing services for individuals infected or affected by HIV/AIDS in the study region[6]. Organisations whose services targeted children aged 0- 8 years were invited to nominate caregiver - and child respondents.

Organisations fell into two categories:

1)   'large organisations': These included umbrella and multifaceted agencies which coordinate and/or implement several diverse programs.

---

[6] Some organisations did not meet the criteria for participating in the study. However, interviews with all representatives were included in data gathering. Representatives from all organisations were able to provide information about 'macro' issues affecting young children even when they were not catering to this population.

2)   'small organisations': These included individuals or agents who were engaged in the delivery of one or a few services with similar foci.

Caregivers included individuals who were providing direct care to children infected or affected by HIV/ AIDS. Caregivers were situated in non-community based settings, safety houses and residential settings. The latter group were living in their own homes. They tended to be relatives or have other close connections with the children in their care.

Children included in the study were aged from 0- 9 years. They were identified by caregivers and others as being infected or affected by HIV/AIDS. Most children were orphans or had mothers who were known to be HIV positive or were not able to care for the children for other reasons. Interviews were held with 12 children. Some of these were known to be HIV positive.

Interview procedures

Interview questions were developed from the literature and addressed perceived gaps in information. Representatives from organisations were given the opportunity to comment on interview questions prior to the study. Minor adjustments were made following this feedback (see Appendix I).

Research assistants (RAs) were recruited who had experience working with families and children and who were fluent in the language of the participants. The RAs did not have in-depth expertise in the area of early childhood development. In this way they were deemed to be less likely to make comparisons with a set of (early childhood development) norms and thus to manipulate responses (consciously or subliminally) through body language or other signals.

The RAs were given training in interview techniques. Training included orientation to the study, review of interview techniques and common issues associated with interviewing children and others, observations of interviews with sample participants, post observation debriefing sessions and trialling the interview questions in simulated situations.

RAs attempted to visit each participating service at least twice in order to establish relationships prior to formal interviews[7].

Interviews with caregivers took place in the language of the respondent which was a first or second language of the interviewers. Audio recorders were used during interviews when permission was granted by the respondent.(It was deemed inappropriate to use audio recorders for children's interviews because of their distracting nature) .

Children were interviewed in their first language and in their own familiar surroundings . RAs spent some time observing and/or playing with children prior to the 'interview'. Children were given 'tools'-

---

[7]This was not always possible, especially in residential settings. In these cases RAs spent time with the interviewees in informal discussion prior to addressing the interview questions. In several instances, RAs participated in care-giving activities during their visits as a way to counter the notion of an interview hierarchy.

crayons, markers and paper and asked to draw pictures during the course of the interview. Younger children and those who were not familiar with writing implements were given 'play-dough' and invited to make sculptures as they talked with interviewers. Pictures and sculptures were collected with permission of the child. The tools were left at the setting to be shared with the other children.

Interview responses were translated into English by RAs and were transcribed by a third party[8].

Validation of findings

Participating organisational representatives, ministry officials and other interested parties were invited to a feedback session during which collated findings from the interviews were presented. Participants were given the opportunity to comment, to enhance, and/or to qualify the data presented. Comments were recorded by a third party.

Analyses

Data was analysed in two ways. Firstly data was categorised according to the interview questions. The questions reflect the international literature about the factors associated with long-term health and well-being for children and adults. These factors constitute a typography of human rights and needs which moves from survival needs through to conditions for freedom of choice (See Box 1). Question development was also influenced by the notion that there are global (universal) attributes which transcend context and contribute to organisational functioning. Five characteristics have been correlated to effective early childhood programs on a global scale. These are listed in Box 2.

Secondly, data was analysed for 'grounded' findings. All transcripts, including the comments from the feedback session, were run through a computer program which assists in qualitative data analysis (QSR Nvivo). This program enables provision of search categories and reveals sets and patterns which may not have been anticipated by the research design (Gahan & Hannibal, 1999; Hiner, 2000; Qualitative Solutions and Research Pty Ltd, 1997).

FINDINGS

Services available for target population in the study region

Respondents were able to provide a diverse list of programs and services for OVCs and their families operating in the study region. The gamut reflected every level of the *typography of human rights and needs* (see Box 1*)*. However all respondents reported that the extent to which coverage extended to all of those who would and could benefit from the programs and services was unknown.

---

[8] It is acknowledged that some nuances and meanings might have been lost during translation processes. However this was deemed to be worth the risk. Relying on English speakers only would have eliminated many appropriate respondents from the study.

Two Centres in the study (A and B) were developed specifically for young children. Other than this, very few programs specifically targeted the 0-8 year population.

However many programs were deemed to have an indirect effect on young children through assistance to relatives, caregivers and/or siblings. For example, if school age siblings were accessing a lunch program, the food at home could be given to the young child. Other services such as support groups for mothers who are HIV positive and home based care programs were similarly seen to be providing indirect benefits to young children.

How services are developed

Larger organisations report having an infrastructure that allows them to assess needs and develop services. Most organisations appear to have the grass roots communication structures and policy-making ability to assess changing needs and establish services to meet those needs. Services targeting young children were not generally identified as a priority need or were seen to be 'covered' through programs for caregivers.

One small organisation did target this population and had scrutinised their community (through door to door interviews and community meetings) to identify children in need of assistance.

Services reported to be available in the study region addressed all levels of the typography of human rights and needs (including survival, health, well-being, education and support for life-choice). However, respondents reported that many services could be expanded and other needed services could be developed if funding and other supports were available to them.

Data base of services

At least one organisation keeps a national database of OVCs, including the supports which are provided for these children. The Ministry of Women's Affairs and Child Welfare also keep records. However a centralised system and monitoring process to determine existing, past and potential members for this database does not appear to be available. It is not known if various databases contain information about the same children. It is not known what percentage of appropriate children for the database has been included or what percentage of OVCs is receiving the support they need. Specific information about 0-8 year old OVCs is not readily available.

Programs available

The programs currently operating in the study region included:

<u>Survival programs</u>

- Needs assessment by community volunteers (followed by distribution of goods and services to identified needy families and/or community groups);

- Safe homes: OVCs can live here temporarily. Officially registered safe homes receive N$10 per day per child. Monitoring is informal (i.e. neighbors may report incidences. There is no formal process for de-registration) ;

- Home based visiting;

- Soup kitchens: lunches for school children;

- Emergency and temporary accommodation for children;

- Special 'Fete' days when families can receive donated goods (3 times per year);

- Fostering of babies when they have nowhere else to go.

<u>Health programs</u>

- Vouchers for purchasing anti-retroviral and other medications;

- Health services;

- Support with maintaining medication schedules;

- Nutrition programs;

- Exercise and massages;

- Accessibility and support for HIV/AIDS testing, including counselling, and other support services for those found to be HIV positive;

- Dissemination of documents to access health and medical services.

<u>Programs aimed at well-being, psychosocial development, family and community connections</u>

- Home based visits;

- Counselling for 0-18 year old OVCs including a weekly support group (NOTE: Children aged 0-8years do not access support groups. Instead they attend the mother support group with their mothers.);

- Support groups for infected adults and caregivers;

- Support for residential (relative) care in the community;

- Opportunities to meet and interact with others in an informal way;

- Promotion of adoption for orphans;

- Counselling for pregnant women.

Formal education and training programs

- Training for community volunteers;

- Training for home based visitors;

- Day-care preschool program, providing food and medicine;

- Camps for older children;

- After school tutoring;

- Training for caregivers (including workshops on *Building Resilience In Children Affected By HIV/AIDS; Home Based Family Care In Namibia; How To Start A Support Group*);

- School fee vouchers;

- Provision of school uniforms.

Freedom of expression, choice and movement

- Income generating projects for infected mothers (Young children often accompany the mothers, but no activities are organised for the children);

- Bursaries for exceptional children to attend secondary school;

- Raising awareness about HIV/AIDS including advocacy for acceptance of HIV positive children and their mothers.

- Children in residential settings who had access to day programs such as school lunch program and day care program, which serves meals were not experiencing these deficiencies.

How children access services and programs

Information about services available to OVCs is disseminated through community agents such as Churches, schools and NGOs, government departments, support groups, community volunteers, door-to-door visits, and general public awareness (radio, posters, brochures) and by word of mouth.

In one case the centre became known when it set up in a community and was able to take in children who appeared at the door. Now it is full and provides services according to priority criteria determined by the organisation: Many children who would benefit remain unable to access this service. The centre is currently looking for ways to expand its delivery to accommodate the numbers presenting themselves.

The belief that there may be many OVCs who are not known, not registered or not accessing services was reported by all respondents.

One of the small organisations reported that they are aware of the needs of the 0-8 year old population in their own (small) geographical location.

We think we know about them all… went door to door in this area – had community meeting

Director of small organisation

Monitoring and quality of service provision and delivery

No formal monitoring of quality of service provision was identified during this study. Organisations reported that informal monitoring took place and/or that remarks by neighbors would sometimes alert them to distressful situations for their children.

Researchers used observations and interview data to assess the extent to which services were meeting established criteria for effective early childhood programs (see Box 2 above) These are described as follows:

1) Programs are community driven and highly participatory

Organisations and centres appeared to be community driven: That is, they were based on needs identified in and from the community, were situated where needs were prevalent and were run by or included staff and volunteers from the community and from the client population.

In Centre B the impetus and management of the service had emanated from a source outside the community (an international organisation). Management and staff did not include community representatives.[9]

2) Programs emphasise a wide diversity of areas concerning children's health and well-being

Centre A was a small organisation which ran multi service programs including home based visiting, support groups for mothers, income generation (in planning stages) and links with several other organisations. Children in the centre interacted in their community but were branded as being 'from the AIDS house'. It was reported that some neighbourhood children had been told not to play with the centre children because of this stigma. A four-year-old had been barred from the local kindergarten because of his HIV positive status.

Centre B focussed primarily on providing an 'educational' program' for 3-6 year olds. This was supplemented by serving nutritious meals, organising for health checks, occasional visits by doctors, and distribution of prescribed medicines for the children. This organisation did not focus on family support or related services nor was it linked to schools or other community services at the time of the study.

Centre C was based within the community. Children attended community schools. There ap peared to be linkages with other social service providers. Volunteers from NGOs came on an adhoc basis to interact with children. A large organisation had an association with this centre, including referrals and placement of children. Monitoring was not observed but a representative from the large organisation reported that they would respond if complaints were made. (The centre reported having more than the allotted capacity of children, because the children had no-where else to go.) School aged children at this centre appeared to mingle with non-OVCs in the community.

Centre D had contacts with schools, training programs and health services. The Centre con tained homes within a large compound, behind a security gate. Children did not mingle with non-OVCs in the neighbourhood.

Centre E is a decentralised large organisation which runs many programs. Children in residen-tial homes associated with Centre E were integrated in their neighbourhoods and communities and were accessing health and nutrition programs through the large organisation.

3)   Programs emphasise strategic communications for awareness rising

The large organisations were highly committed to this activity. Numerous brochures and post ers were produced and disseminated widely. Workshops and training packages were devel oped for diverse participants. Books were published and distributed through a variety of outlets. Income generation projects served double purposes of raising awareness and raising funds (for example the production of beaded AIDS brooches and story books for children).

Centre A played an active role in raising awareness about the needs of infected and affected individuals and children. Radio and print media were used to promote positive messages about these issues. Community meetings were held to discuss the importance of not rejecting HIV positive people and families. Centre B reported on their success with *'flag days'* whereby people celebrate the anniversary of the day they become aware of their HIV positive status and vow to

---

[9] It was reported that this issue was being reviewed and programs to take on volunteers or trainees from the community were being discussed.

live positively with the disease. They also engage in small scale awareness raising:

We… sensitised people in the area. We had community meetings. We even went from door-to-door. That's why we never have a burglary, because (everyone) knows we are the "AIDS-house". Blankets can be outside for a week.

Director, small organisation

Centre B, Centre C, Centre D and the residential houses did not appear to engage in awareness raising activities. Centre E is very active and has a strong infrastructure which supports awareness raising about all facets of HIV/AIDS.

4) Programs have links to community programs including schools

One large organisation reported having exceptionally close relations with health and educational agents and was thus able to provide services for its registered clients in an effective and efficient manner. All organisations expressed a desire to increase inter-agency linkages and to develop vehicles for information- sharing and referrals, but time and coordination needed for this was not deemed to be a priority in light of service-oriented needs.

One safe house identified links with schools. All safe houses reported linkages with health and social service providers.

Many caregivers in residential houses were receiving assistance from Centre E. However, many caregivers reported feeling unconnected. Some were in conflict with community services such as municipalities and schools who were making funding claims upon them. Many respondents in residential houses reported that they could not access adequate health services and/or did not appear to know where to seek assistance for the children in their care.

The school is always threatening with letters to pay the school fees otherwise the children will be out of school. The municipality is also threatening with the payment of the house, water and electricity

Caregiver in residential house (rh)

need school fees and schoolbooks because they are threatening from the school

Caregiver in rh

She is not well informed… she does not know where to seek help, who to talk to and how to find solutions to her problems.

RA comments on caregiver in rh

5)	Programs provide training opportunities for sustainability

The stability of infrastructures to ensure sustainability of current levels of service delivery and to facilitate the development of new programs as needs emerge was not evident in all situations.

At one Centre, a sustainable infrastructure was in place. This service had been operating for several decades. The infrastructure would protect service continuity beyond the presence of anyone individual such as the Head/Director .

At another Centre, the commitment of one individual was the driving force behind service development and delivery. The absence of this individual could result in program closure.

The majority of caregivers in residential houses (all but 2) reported having no backup should they become ill or unable to care for the child (ren) in their care. This was a source of grave concern to many caregivers.

 As long as I am alive everything will go well, but what will happen to them if I pass away one day?

Elderly caregiver in rh

Training

One large organisation reported a training (and advancement) program for their staff. Most respondents in this study were not engaging in professional development activities. Caregivers in safe houses were aware that organisations were offering workshops/training in relevant topics, but only one respondent reported having attended any such program. In one safe house, turnover of caregivers was rapid. Caregivers seemed to have no experience or preferred background for the position. Training did not seem to be accessible due to lack of awareness, lack of time and/or lack of interest/ commitment by some workers at this safehouse.

FUNDING ISSUES

Sources of funds

Large and small organisations reported that their funding relied heavily on donations, usually from NGOs, Churches, and individuals.

Fundraising events, income generation projects and Ministry assistance for direct support to orphans (when accessed) were also mentioned as sources of funds. Community donations, including free rent in two cases, were a major source of funds

Children in safe houses who are registered with the Ministry of Women's Affairs and Child Welfare receive N$10 per day, paid to safe house operators. The director of one safe house explained that the rules for receiving funding were not comprehensive because many needy children who were not 'officially' orphans remained ineligible. Further, requirements for accessing the funds were reported to be rigid and complex. For these reasons at least one centre in the study was not accessing this source of funding [10].

Security of funding

Large organisations who reported diverse sources of income were confident of stability of funding. All organisations stated that they were continually seeking additional sources of income to enhance existing services and to develop new programs. Many current programs depended upon donations. Fundraising was reported to be increasingly competitive, and constant seeking of new sources was needed[11].

We get support from the State with food, clothing, shelter. But your own initiative is important.

Caregiver in safe house (sh)

This house belongs to the church. We were given up to end of this month to buy this house. Otherwise we will have to move out. But we think a door will open for us soon.

Director of small organisation

Funding needs

Small organisations and residential caregivers identified funding as a major concern in their ability to provide care for the children.

At least one small organisation was facing a deadline for funds and was under threat of losing their accommodation. Caregivers in safe houses reported that lack of funds was a hardship for them. The lack of or inadequacy of caregivers' salaries was a source of distress, including family conflict.

ZZ

We need more donations from individuals and organisations

Director of small organisation

---

[10] Where funds were being received, there appeared to be little monitoring by the source, nor was there evidence that the receiving child was benefiting directly from this funding. Analyses of policies such as this one lay outside of the parameters of the study. Further investigation of this issue is called for

[11] Surprisingly, no organisation mentioned corporate donations as a source of funds. The potential to garner corporate support for programs needs to be explored.

We live from day to day – we take things as they come

Director of small organisation

The majority of Residential caregivers reported deprivations due to lack of funding and support. Concerns included threats from schools, municipalities and others because of outstanding debts. Lack of funds for school uniforms, for adequate food, for 'nice clothes, and for goods which would keep children entertained such as a television and bicycle.'

I have to pay school fees and buy clothes for the children. The pension fund money is not enough. I need a television for the children and.. the boy needs a bicycle. I do not know what the future will bring…One day the children will go to a secondary school and life is very expensive out there.

Caregiver in rh

I do not receive any kind of payment to take care of him. I only depend on my pension and help from my daughter.

Caregiver in rh

I am a very old lady and I only depend on my pension money... I do not get any help or support from anyone.

Caregiver in rh

The only problem is to pay for water & electricity. Without my daughter's help I won't be able to maintain our house

Caregiver in rh

I have financial problems; if any one can help me with money to take care of this child I will be glad.

Caregiver in rh

It will be good for me if the children get help with food and financial support.

Caregiver in rh

I need help in the form of clothing, blankets and other things.

Caregiver in rh

I (need) assistance with money, food and clothing.

Caregiver in rh

RAs reported that some residential caregivers associated the interview with potential donations. For this reason some respondents may have exaggerated their funding needs. However observations by members of the research team did confirm impoverished situations for children including lack of food, lack of variety in food, lack of adequate clothing, lack of warm bedding, lack of vitamins and medication, lack of space, including adequate sleeping facilities, and other needs.

The hardest thing for me is that we get no privacy: We are sleeping with the children...

Caregiver in sh

B. is a very old lady. She is the only breadwinner at her house.... I interviewed her at her house. The house is really not in good condition. It is empty . There is nothing in her house. The house is very old and the paint is also falling off.

The place was not really quiet or private...She had a lot of complaints and could not stop talking about the problems that she was faced with.

RA observations re rh

G. is also like the other participants thinking that I am a representative of a donor. Nonetheless she seems to be very honest. She is very sick, she is coughing. Her feet are swollen and she is having wounds on the parts of the body which are exposed.... She is really very poor, there is not even a single chair, and we were sitting on stones outside...The environment is not conducive for children. It is dirty, the pots are lying around and they are dirty.

RA observations re rh

Children's rights and needs

For participants in the study, children's rights, needs and their quality of life were assessed through interviews (with children, caregivers, and organisation director) and through observations by researchers[12].

---

[12] The limitations of drawing conclusions from this form of data gathering are acknowledged. It is recommended that empirical assessments of the state of health and well-being for children and their caregivers be undertaken.

Survival

While the majority of children in the study appeared to be having consistent or appropriate access to food and medicine, in one safe house and in several residential houses living conditions were observed or reported to be impoverished and/or below community standards, including inadequate space, bedding, and food. Some children did not meet community standards of cleanliness. Some unhygienic practices (such as sharing eating utensils amongst sick children) were observed. Children in residential settings were most needy in terms of survival and health needs.

The place is not hygienically clean. The children are sometimes fed with one spoon. The toddler's nappies are not changed regularly, because there is not enough manpower. The toddlers can also not nap, especially after school, because the children are too many for three rooms.

Observation by RA re sh

.Sometimes we spend a day without eating till my daughter comes home from work and gives us something to eat.

Caregiver in rh

Most of the time they never eat breakfast.

Caregiver in rh

Their clothes are torn and they are getting cold during winter and they are also barefoot.

Caregiver in rh

Most of the time they don't eat breakfast, lunch and most meals during the weekends.

Caregiver in rh

Sometimes we don't have electricity, or bread to take to school.

Child in rh, age 8

Despite this, none of the children in the study were deemed to be living in conditions that threatened their survival.

Health and well-being

Health status

A percentage of children in this study were suspected or known to be HIV positive. Some children were on medication. A number of children appeared to be very ill and uncomfortable which was presumed to be caused by medication (antiretrovirals).

Space for sleeping, changes of nappies and adequate food provision for very young babies was not provided in one safe home. Young children were observed being disturbed in their sleep and/or bullied by older children at this setting. Hygiene practices were not being followed on the day of the interview. For example all children (some obviously very ill) were using the same spoon.

Despite this, the majority of the children included in this study appeared to be clean and adequately nourished.

> S. is very shy and withdrawn…. She has skin rashes all over her body. Her eyes are reddish and she is quite thin for her age…She was well dressed and looked clean.
>
> RA observations on child in sh

> J. appears too small for 6 years, but clean.
>
> RA observations on child in sh

In one residential house the children appeared stunted and malnourished. They had recently joined a program at a large organisation and may now be receiving food more regularly.

> D. was not able to respond well to the interview. She's very withdrawn and shy. One can really see that she is living in a poverty stricken house. Her clothing was not well, especially regarding the weather conditions on this day. She was too underdressed. She also looked underfed. For a child of seven years, she was very small. She looks more like a four year old.
>
> Observation by RA re child in rh

Well-being

> *They always get shocked when they are removed from their parents however bad the home was…It feels like death.*
>
> Caregiver in sh

Researchers observed symptoms associated with trauma, depression and lack of bonding/attachment in young children[13]. No child in this study had been psychologically assessed nor were they accessing formal counselling of any sort.

Access to experiences which address psychosocial needs such as consistency in caretaking appeared to be unmet for many of the children in the study. In one safe house, the time, space and attention paid to the youngest children (aged 0- 5 years) were observed to be inadequate in many ways[14].

---

[13] No formal testing of mental health was conducted during this study. Comments are based on observed behaviours including clinging to strangers, lack of eye contact, poor attention span, lack of affect, lack of energy, withdrawal or reluctance to interact with adults and/or peers.

[14] Testing of this variable was not included in the study. Findings are based on reports from caregivers and children and on observations of up to several hours and/or across several days of children in their settings.

Interviewers noted clinging and other behaviors associated with feelings of loneliness, trauma and depression in a number of children at safe houses. This could be associated with caregiver turnover which constrains bonding experiences for young children. The clinging behaviors were not apparent in the safe house where caregivers had been employed for long periods of time.

Children's daily routines described by caregivers in all settings were similar. These included eating, bathing, taking medicines and playing outside (or watching TV in some cases). Age-appropriate toys and play materials were not observed in safe houses or residential houses. Young children were not observed to be engaged in activities which are associated with cognitive and psychosocial development. Individual attention for babies, two-way interactions between children and adults or older children, cooperative group play, exposure to stimulating and challenging experiences through a variety of materials and activities, opportunities for large muscle development, opportunities for quiet, and reflective experiences were not observed during visits to houses.

Experiences associated with school readiness such as talking, looking at written symbols, singing, counting and similar activities were not witnessed during the study period.

A number of children reported that they had 'friends' in their safe houses. Caring and positive interactions between older and younger children was observed in some safe houses when the older children returned from school. However quality time with adults whereby two-way interactions, communication and 'teaching' are prevalent was not observed throughout the study period. In response to questions about providing developmental experiences for children, caregivers gave answers such as:

> *We are not trained to be preschool teachers.*
>
> Caregiver in sh
>
> *We would like to take them to the park but we have no transport.*
>
> Caregiver in sh
>
> *There is nothing positive about this place.*
>
> Caregiver in sh
>
> *We rarely have time to read (play with) them.*
>
> Caregiver in sh
>
> *(All I can do is) walk around the block with the child – or play games when they are upset – We definitely need a psychiatrist.*
>
> Caregiver in sh

Children observed at the day care program (Centre B) were the exception. At this centre, age-appropriate, stimulating experiences were being provided for the 37 children enrolled (including child participants in this study).

The majority of children in the study seemed to lack a sense of their place and history. Many children (and caregivers) did not know about their background:

> K was brought by the police. His parents are in prison. He is from
> Okahandja. The police never came back to inform him about anything

concerning his family.

Caregiver in sh re child aged 6

J came when he was only 1year old. He lost his mom during childbirth. He was brought by the social workers and we've heard nothing about his relatives since.

Caregiver in sh re child aged 4

F came from hospital. He was 5 months. He was born in Katima. His mother was positive. He came as Baby F; no mother's name, nothing. No details of family. Only this year did we find out his surname.

Caregiver in sh re child aged 2 1/2.

Narratives by children often revealed a sense of confusion and/or rejection:
They put my father in a big hole and now I live here.

Child in sh

Do you know who brought you here? *No.*

Child in sh, aged 6

He changed houses in the compound a short while ago. It seems as if he does not remember anything before that.

RA about child aged 5.

He says he is 3 years, his friend says he is 5. The caregiver says he is 5.

RA

I believe he is not well informed about himself. He does not know his own age.

RA re child in sh

Some children obviously believed that something wrong with them had resulted in their current predicament and/or they held other simplistic views about their situation:
My mother is in Owamaboland. She doesn't want me to live there. (Why not?)
I don't know.

Child in sh

My mother does not want me anymore.

Child in sh

Why are you here? *I am sick.*

Child in sh, aged 5

Other children had a grasp of their situation:
My mother and father died because they have AIDS.

Child in sh

*"Aunty" brought me with my mother and my sister .Where are they now?:
They are in Rehoboth.*

Child in sh

Information about and access to resources for stimulating cognitive, emotional and psychosocial development in young children was deemed to be a need for caregivers and children in this study[15]. Access to counselling and other therapies to overcome disruption and trauma in the children's lives could have positive effects on their current and future health and well-being.

Formal *Education/Training*

The children make progress. The schools also give reports that the children are improving.

Caregiver in sh

(Sometimes) children are sent back from school because of outstanding school fees.

Caregiver in rh

Problems with accessing school fees and school uniforms were identified by several residential caregivers. A number of others were accessing school uniforms and vouchers for school fees from a large organisation. This was mentioned as being invaluable to those who were benefitting from the program.

At least two children in residential homes were beyond school age and had never attended any educational institution.

Children in safe homes appeared to be able to access the commodities for school (uniforms and fees). One child of school age in a safe house was not attending school but the caregiver stated that this was because she was too sick to travel and that a school closer to the house was being sought.

Space and assistance for studying (attending to homework and other educational activities) was deemed to be a need in all situations (except for Centre D where space and designated time for 'homework' was available).

Organised activities for young children which are associated with cognitive development (interacting with materials, pre-literacy and pre-numeracy experiences) took place in Centre B. As noted above, these types of activities were not observed or reported as being available for the children who did not attend that Centre.

---

[15] Some excellent resources have been developed by large organisations along these lines, notably *Building Resilience In Children Affected By HIV/AIDS; Home Based Family Care In Namibia; How To Start A Support Group (CAA). However only* one caregiver in the study reported being unable to access training opportunities.

Freedom of expression, choice and movement

For young children these factors are associated with 'normalcy' and can be assessed by examining the visions that they have for their futures (reflecting a perceived ability to achieve these visions).

Normalcy

Children in residential houses appeared to have their psychosocial needs met to a greater extent than other children: love, attachment, consistency, 'normalcy', a sense of their own history and family ties and integration within their communities were most apparent in these situations. Residential caregivers however tended to be in their senior years and reported illness, exhaustion and constant worry over finances and/or over how the children would fare in the future. Children in residential settings were also deemed to be most *needy* in terms of health needs:

> *I really can't provide decent clothing and good food for (child).Sometimes we even spent a day without eating till my daughter comes home from work and gives us something to eat*
>
> Caregiver in rh

In answer to the question,' *what are the current needs of the children in your care?'* Residential caregivers identified the following:

Children need :

> *..funds for paying the school fees, food, clothes, hospital if they are sick as well as outstanding balance for the house and water and electricity.*
> *.clothing and shoes. financial support. better living and accommodation.*
> *...clothes: (large organisation) is only sometimes providing clothes, otherwise, they are wearing torn clothes.*
> *...school fees and books are a big problem...and we don't have a TV at home.*
> *... food. the food (here) is not enough and they are eating only one type of food.*
> *..clothes..*
> *..space. They are sharing the sleeping room with their uncles, aunts and parents and it's difficult to study under this situation.*
>
> Caregivers in rh

Caregivers in safe houses often expressed feelings of love for the children. However conditions such as overwork, high ratios of children to caregiver, caregiver illness and stigma attached to living in a safe house were seen to increase turnover and/or inconsistencies in care which are associated with stress and distress in children.

In answer to the question, *what are the current needs of the children in your care?* Caregivers in safe houses identified the following:

Children need:

...A family must be involved and they need a social life.

..support to build confidence to themselves and acceptance.

.. a better environment for studying.

... a pre-school teacher.

.. .definitely, a psychologist.

Caregivers in sh

In one non-community based safe house, consistency of caregiving and of peer-group interaction was high. The children in the house, however, were isolated within their compound, did not interact with non-OVCs (except at school) and seemed constrained in opportunities to be part of a 'normal' community life. The fact that some children had remained in the safe house into adulthood reflects their sense of non-inclusion into society.

> *They don't want to be told that they are in an orphanage (sic)...Even if an orphanage is trying to offer the basic needs to cover all the needs. The children at the orphanage are missing out on real family life. When the children complete matric they feel insecure. Because they do not know what the future looks like....*

Caregiver in non-community based sh

Visions of the future

While it might be expected that images of adulthood have been tainted by experiences with sickness and death for children in this study, for the most part children answered the question *'What do you want to be?'* in age-appropriate ways. Responses seemed related to life experience and included being doctors who could cure people, police workers who would 'kill' or arrest bad people, and on several occasions, 'shovellers' or others who put people in the ground. A church related future was envisioned by some children. In all cases, responses did not reflect despair or a sense of impending death.

> *(I want to be) a doctor. To operate people.*

> *I want to become a doctor so that I can heal sick people so they won't die and... they can return home to their families.*

> *I want to be a Christian, to pray everyday and to go to church.*

I want to become a soldier…because a soldier took Jesus and put him on the cross.

I want to become a policeman and shoot the children (sic) and drive away.

I want to work with shovels and cleaning the house when people die.
I will clean the yard, shovelling.

Children

A number of children have visions of material wealth for themselves.

 I want to work and earn a lot of money to be rich and buy a lot of things and many things to eat…. buy a lot of furniture and a big house.

I want to buy clothes.
I want to work for company and buy myself a big house and a lot of FOOD.
I want to buy a house and stay with my children.
I want a BMW... a big one!

Children

Positive experiences of children

While many deprivations were noted, nearly all caregivers believed that the children were currently in the best situation possible under the circumstances.

A number of encouraging statements were made about children by caregivers in all situations:

When they came here they seemed to have no hope – you did not believe that they would wake up in the morning - but now most of them are well – they are fine. They put a smile on my face.

I thought we were going to bury M (child aged 6 months) but there she is – I think that her mother's death gave her motivations!

We cannot replace family but we give them love and care.

At least they are healthy under this difficult situation. And they have a room.

The children come from difficult circumstances. Now they have their own bed. They sit at the table with a Mummy. They have shelter.

The children they have a place to sleep and eat, they have a home.

Some of these children have nothing, nobody… They are better off here.

I think they get everything…I take them to the swimming pool. We buy toys.

This is a very stable situation.
There is no better place for the children.

Caregivers in safe houses

The children themselves also expressed acceptance or happiness with the situation

I like it here. I get macaroni.

Child in sh

The food is good. Sometimes we have ice cream and apples. We also play around with toys and games.

Child in sh

We play with our friends. Aunty T (the caregiver) gives us nice things like lolli-pops. We play around the house.

Child in sh

I like playing with the children. I like cleaning our rooms.

Child in sh

I like playing with friends…The bread is nice.

Child in sh

(I like) playing …when (grandma) tells me stories.. watching TV at neighbours. We eat nice food.

Child in rh

(I like) my (siblings).(He has four siblings).

Child in rh

My mom (sic) takes care of me. She loosens my hair and washes the clothes. She cleans the home. She gives me food. We eat bread. (There are) birthdays and Christmas. We watch TV and video. We have porridge and chocolates.

Child in rh

Observations by researchers included positive aspects of children's experiences.

The children were clean and appropriately fed. The older children coming from school seemed happy.

RA re children in sh

B. (age 9) appeared collected and happy. He was very open-minded and confident. He seems to have accepted his situation quite well. He also seemed to understand that his parents died and this Home was the only other place he could go. He spoke in English.

RA re child in rh

D. (age 5) was obviously well looked after, although for his age his speech was poor.

RA re child in sh

W. (age 5) is a very outspoken little boy. He can express himself well and he is very talkative. He is friendly and smiles a lot. . He has a high level of communication and he seems very healthy although he looks very small for his age, and he did not look too clean...

RA re child in rh

J (age 4) is a very friendly little girl. She is not shy at all. Her level of communication is good and she was able to respond well. She looked healthy and clean. She smiles a lot and could express herself well.

RA re child in rh

Children who attended the day care centre and remained in residential homes had many advantages over other children. They were assured good nourishment and assistance with medical needs. Their residential caregivers were given respite during 'school' hours. They interacted with other children who attended the centre and were not stigmatised by their situation. The day care centre (Centre B) also provided stimulating group experiences appropriate to the age of the children. This would assist with integration and achievement when the children entered the public school system.

Children in residential homes who were school age and accessing the programs of the large organisation (lunch and after school tutoring) were similarly advantaged. These programs alleviated stress for residential caregivers regarding food for the children. These children also received uniforms, other clothes and goods such as blankets from the organisation.

(Large organisation) is sometimes providing clothes… otherwise they are wearing torn clothes.

Caregiver in rh

I am assisted by the support from (large organisation) - the meals they are offering during week days to children, the food, blankets and clothes that they give.

Caregiver in rh

They get schoolbooks and school uniforms from (large organisation).

Caregiver in rh

The children are getting lunch during weekdays from (large organisation).

Caregiver in rh

*Luckily the (large organisation) is providing meals to the young children and some-
time school uniforms.*

Caregiver in rh

Children's' Stories

*I brought up J's mother. When she passed away because of HIV/AIDS, I brought up J and her
brother. They have both been with me since birth. They are like my own children and even if I
passed away, J will stay with my cousin who is also part of the family… They help with little tasks at
home. They play with their friends outside. B. most of the time plays soccer with friends J. plays
with dolls made out of materials, sometimes with her friends just outside or sometimes alone at
home. They get sent to the shop to buy things like bread, milk and sugar etc… They don't have toys
like balls or bicycle to play with. They don't always have all the meals per day . There is not enough
space for them to play... My husband died four years ago and my own son died two years ago. I
still have to pay for the house, water and electricity. I have to pay school fees and buy clothes for
the children and the pension fund money is not enough. They get school uniforms from (large
organisation)....I do not know what the future will bring for them because; one day the children
have to go to a secondary school and life is very expensive out there… They give me light everyday…..*

Caregiver in rh

During the interview I witnessed the respondent telling the boy to stop playing in the street. He told her
that one day when he grows up he is going to play in the national team. He will also go abroad and
play soccer there and get a lot of money. His grandmother will see him on television and he will be well
known. He will also buy his grandmother a big house in Klein Windhoek, like Frank Fredericks, and a
television. ..The respondent is obviously very attached to the children and you can see how much she
enjoys it when they are telling her their dreams and promises.

RA observation of caregiver above

*Joyce and John are brother and sister. They came here four years ago. They were very neglected –
had 'scars' and suffering from malnutrition. No parent visited for two year; by coincidence, a worker
here recognized the children. We started looking for the parents. We found that they were not drinking
anymore. The situation has improved a lot. They did not know where the children were. But they now
visit their parents during weekends. Things are going well for them. But their parents have to get their
own accommodation before they can go to them….*

Caregiver in sh

My uncle brought us here when my mom was in the hospital. At first he used to visit us, but now we don't see him anymore. We cannot stay with our mom because there is no food at home. She only comes to visit us here.

Child in sh, aged 8

Teacher C brought me here when my mom died.. My father also died and all my relatives died. Nobody (that I knew) came with me. My mom used to play netball with the other people and she always won…. The caregivers take care of me. I like playing with toys and also with the other children. I also like cleaning our rooms. D. is my best friend, she also lives here. I don't like S (who lives in house). H beats and bites the children (quoted earlier). He is very messy. I want to become a doctor so that I can heal sick people so they won't die and they can return home to their families. (quoted earlier)

Child in sh, aged 6

J. came when he was only 1year old. He lost his mom during childbirth. He was brought by the social workers and we've heard nothing about his relatives since. There is no other place he can go and there is no way he can be reunited with his family. (quoted earlier)

Caregiver in sh

Stephan came from hospital. He was 5 months. His mother was positive. He came with no mother's name, no details of family, nothing. He is positive but is not active. We don't tell the other children that he has HIV. But we told the others that when he is bleeding; don't touch it as he has a disease in his blood. He is awaiting adoption. He has been asking about his mother. He also wants to be taken out for weekends. He will now go out for outings. His HIV is not active yet. He might live up to 15 years.

Caregiver in sh

Caregiver's rights and needs

Young children's survival, health, well-being and access to services and to experiences which allow them to fulfill their potential are dependent upon the adults who are available to provide protection, care and nurturance. When caregivers are incapacitated or unavailable to children because of illness, stress, financial concerns or other reasons, the care of the children will be affected.

For these reasons this study included investigations of the experiences and conditions experienced by caregivers of OVCs in the study region. Findings are reported according to the typography of human rights and needs (See Box 1). Caregivers' experiences are categorised according to the situation: caregiving in a residential house or caregiving in a safe house. Experiences however are shown to be unique for each situation. Generalisability by these categories alone is not appropriate or possible.

Survival

<u>Residential caregivers</u>

While some residential caregivers were living in conditions of deprivation, basic conditions for survival were present in all situations. For the most impoverished, the old-age pension appeared to be covering basic needs on a day-to-day basis. For those residential caregivers who accessed assistance for their children in the form of daycare services, school vouchers and school uniforms, lunch programs and donations of clothes, blankets and other goods, life was made substantially more bearable.

<u>Caregivers in safe houses</u>

Basic survival needs were not an issue for caregivers in safe houses. There were no reports of inadequate access to food and shelter.

Health and well-being

<u>Residential caregivers</u>

The majority of caregivers in residential houses reported being ill, tired, badly nourished and/or highly stressed.

> *I do all the cooking and cleaning in the house and during weekends my daughter will help me. My only free time is when he is at school. I do not receive any kind of payment to take care of him. I only depend on my pension and help from my daughter. (quoted earlier)*
>
> Caregiver in rh

> *I am a very old lady and I only depend on my pension money... I do not get any help or support from anyone. (quoted earlier)*
>
> Caregiver in rh

> *I am an old lady... I have problems with my eyes, I need glasses, but the money is not there. (quoted earlier)*
>
> Caregiver in rh

Concern over financial burdens was prevalent in this population. Residential caregivers were also concerned that as children got older they would need more material goods and/or become more difficult to 'discipline'. Anxiety was expressed about the ability to continue caregiving, to meet future financial needs and about what will happen when they pass away.

> *.... My pension is not enough for both of us.*
> *Too many children to take care of on a pension – not enough food or goods for all.*

(I worry about)..funds for paying the school fees, food, clothes, hospital if they are sick as well as outstanding balance for the house and water and electricity.

> *As long as I am alive every thing will go well, but what will happen to them if I pass away one day? (quoted earlier)*
>
> Caregivers in rh

Many residential caregivers reported being unable to find a way to increase their income – despite a willingness to do so.

> *(Hardest part is).. the fact that I cannot provide for the children and the fact that I am unemployed...only employment. The fact that I know that I am not going to be around for them for a very long time.*
> *I am buying meat to sell. I could have enough money but all this I spend for every day's necessities, because three of my children are staying with me, my daughter, my two boys as well as my daughter-in-law....It's a very difficult situation.*
>
> *If I can get a sponsor for a project so that I can bake bread and sell or even for ovens and a building. Or even a machine so that I can sew aprons and dresses and sell. Then at least my children's school fees and food will be covered every day.*
>
> *I can't provide because I have nothing....I do not know how and I need em-ployment to provide for these needs* (of the children)
>
> *I find my situation very difficult because I am unemployed. People don't re-spect me. They only misuse me. If I had employment, everything would have been better.*
>
> Caregivers in rh

At least two residential settings did not present health and well-being concerns. They reported being relatively stress-free and proud to be providing a good environment for the children. At one of these homes the caregiver seemed to have only one concern: no television set. She named this as a top priority for the children (implying that basic needs such as food, shelter, clothes, school fees and health items were not lacking at this time).

Caregivers in safe houses

Safe houses presented diverse situations for caregivers (and children).

Sources of worry and stress for caregivers stemmed from worries about children, working and living conditions (in some cases) and ill health of the caregiver (in some cases).

> One of the caregivers herself was sick. She had some kind of sore under her arm that caused

her arm to be swollen. How can anyone work under such a situation? I assume that she also has her own baby at the centre. I wonder how she was able to work with that arm.

RA observations re sh

Some caregivers expressed concern over children's psychological needs which they felt incapable of addressing adequately. The need for discipline and structure for the children was also a concern.

> *We definitely need a psychologist... We used to have a supervisor. He even supervised recreation (for the children)... They need discipline. They don't want routine. They want to continue playing outside. They get naughty... opening taps... opening the hosepipe in the lounge. (For the younger ones) the lack of a pre-school here is also a frustration.*

Caregiver in safe house

> *We need more volunteers for pre-primary children especially for the ones who stay in during holidays. The social worker should organise holiday camps and other social activities.*

Caregiver in safe house

One caregiver reported interference from relatives as a cause of concern:

> *(Relatives) come (to the house) and complain that their children are not clean. They are not thankful.*

Caregiver in safe house

Caregivers expressed stress related to watching children suffer with illness:

Watching the children get sick is the hardest part.

Caregiver in sh

> *I cannot bear to see it when the children get sick – and you can do nothing for them – it makes me depressed. I don't want them to suffer – if such pain could be exchanged I would bear it for them.*

Caregiver in sh

In majority of safe houses included in this study, caregivers were satisfied with their roles. While all mentioned long days of cleaning, cooking, bathing children and similar chores, the majority were not discouraged by the workload. In one safe house the caregivers were HIV positive.[16] In one safehouse caregivers did not receive remuneration. Despite poor health and/or the lack of salary, caregivers reported receiving many rewards for their work and overall satisfaction with their jobs.

> *When children just come in, it is difficult to get them to accept you. When they*

get friendly and they love you, it is really successful!

(The best things are)..to communicate with the children, get acceptance from them, to have that responsibility.
The best reward is the success of the children in your house e.g. when they complete school and get employed.

Life is easy.

I will stay here until I retire.

Caregivers at sh

Caregivers in one safehouse mentioned excursions with children. Caregivers in other situations stated that time or lack of finances and transport prevented regular outings and similar activities.

The need for respite, extra volunteers to care for and/or take the children out, and more time off was mentioned by all categories of caregivers:

Sometimes you just want to drop everything and leave when the children get difficult.

Caregiver in safe house

In one safe house, caregivers seemed very discontent, reporting overwork and poor living conditions. Caregivers in this house reported that daily chores started at 4: 30 am and continued into the evening. Very little or no time was available for personal tasks, for relaxation and/or for interacting with others in the community. Because of the large number of children, lack of space, lack of rest and lack of assistance with many chores, caregivers reported being unable to interact with children on a one-to-one basis. Caregivers received a small salary which appeared to be the major incentive for accepting the position. Despite this long term commitment to the position was not prevalent. Many caregivers left after the first month salary was paid.

Since I first came here I have been waking up everyday at 4 o'clock in the morning, cooking, and sleeping late. It is difficult for me to follow such a program.

Caregiver in sh

It appears that satisfaction with the role of caregiver is related to working conditions. It was also noted that the 'leadership' within the safehouse may be a motivating or demotivating factor for caregivers – along with the feeling of doing a worthwhile task and receiving emotional support for themselves:

I have friends and family who give me moral support .I am happy…I want to motivate

---

[16] One caregiver was observed to be ill and tired during the interview process. She entered hospital during the study period, resulting in the need for a substitute caregiver to enter the house. Other caregivers reported that their HIV possitive status had not affected their ability to care for the children.

others (to speak publicly about their HIV status).

Caregiver at sh

Formal Education/Training

A number of large and small organisations in the study region reported that they offered workshops, training and support groups for home-based caregivers. One large organisation has developed a training program specifically aimed at those taking responsibility for the care of HIV positive children. Participation rates for this (relatively new) program were not assessed.

A small organisation was providing training for families in their home-based visiting scheme:

We have family counselling in the support group. We also provide caregivers and parents with skills to take care of these children.

Director of small organisation

None of the residential (home-based) caregivers in this study reported an awareness of these programs.

Caregivers in safe houses were aware that programs were available but they were not accessing these on a regular basis. One caregiver had recently attended two 'parenting' workshops provided by a large organisation. These were not targeted at special needs for young children or for those who are HIV possitive. Most caregivers in safe houses expressed a desire for training opportunities:

We need more training courses, on communication with the children ...the children should also be trained on rights and responsibilities.

Caregiver in sh

Family counselling and family planning for HIV+ parents were identified by some organisations as a critical need:

We advocate for family planning...There need not be more children in this position if we can prevent it.

Director of small organisation.

Freedom of expression, choice and movement

Residential caregivers

Despite reports of hardships and need for support and assistance to relieve financial burdens, no residential caregiver reported feeling 'trapped' or unhappy with their role in the child's life. All reported that they were offering the best situation for the child. The sentiment of the majority of the caregivers is reflected in the comment below:

What can I say? -If you really love children, there is nothing difficult about taking care of them.

Caregiver in rh

Caregivers in safe houses

The majority of caregivers in safe houses expressed satisfaction with their current situation and the belief that they were performing a valuable role. Every caregiver expressed sentiments similar to the comments below:

In the absence of a family, this house is the best situation for the children.

Caregiver in sh

This job is not for anybody. You must love children against all odds.

Caregiver in sh

Two exceptions were noted. One caregiver was very distressed about her child who was HIV positive living in another region and being taken care of by his grandmother. The caregiver did not have the funds to visit the child when he became ill:

(I)   *need a salary – people do not believe that you are employed but not paid.*
       – when your child is sick you don't even have money to go home.

Caregiver in sh

One caregiver in one safe house reported being unhappy with her position, stating that she preferred work where interactions with children and adults would not be called upon. This caregiver had had no training and was very young (lacking in life experience):

I want to get a job as a domestic.

Caregiver in sh

Positive experiences of Caregivers

Caregiver stories

Residential Caregivers

G. has six children in her home under the age of 9 years. The youngest is 5 days old. Others are 3 years, 6 years, 7 years and there are two 8-year-olds. These are all her grandchildren. One daughter has passed away from HIV/AIDS. G's husband passed away a long time ago. None of her children are working. She is receiving money only from the pension fund. The (large organisation) is providing meals to the young children and sometime school uniforms. First they were giving school fees but now they have stopped. The school is always threatening them with letters that they should pay the school fees; otherwise the children will be out of school. The municipality is also threatening her with the payment of the house, water and electricity. G. buys meat to sell. She could have enough money but all this is spent for every day necessities, because three of her children are staying with her: a

44

daughter, two boys and a daughter-in-law. It's a very difficult situation.

> *I hope we will get help or even my children will get work. One boy is also drinking too much.*

S. has 3 children in her home under the age of 6 years. One boy (N) is an orphan. His mother died of malaria while she was in the north.

> *It was when I received the letter that his mother died, that I asked my brother to take me to the north to get the boy. After a family gathering it was decided that it is best for me to take the boy. By then the boy was very sick and nobody want to take care of him.*
>
> *He was only one year old then. Now he is four years old and there is no place he could go from here...I am a very old lady and I only depend on my pension money. (quoted earlier)*
>
> *I do all the cooking and cleaning in the house and during weekends my daughter will help me. My only free time is when he is at school (a day care centre in the community). I do not receive any kind of payment to take care of him. I only depend on my pension and help from my daughter.... I love children; I could not leave that little boy with strangers that do not love him. He will be with me forever.*

O. is the mother of one baby and two older children. She tested HIV-positive two years ago and she is not healthy. She looked a bit sick but told me that she is now much better. The house was well furnished. She was the only one at home during the interview and it was really comfortable and private.

> *When I started getting sick and weak my mom suggested that(the father's family) may look after the (baby) for a while but they didn't want to...I find my situation very difficult because I am unemployed. People don't respect me, they only misuse me....(Most difficult things are). the fact that I know that I am not going to be around for them for a very long time and the fact I am unemployed. If I had employment, everything would be better. The best thing is the support I get from my Pastor ... when the (older) children return from school. I leave the baby with them for hours..They all play...I need help in the form of clothing, blankets and other things. I can't provide (these things) because I have nothing.*

> *Caregivers in safe house*

After my husband died, Pastor got this job for me in Windhoek. I moved from South Africa to Namibia. I'm here for 18 years at the centre and I love my job. My children grew up there but now they live on their own....I wake up at 5am and prepare the children for school till 6:30 - 7:0. The little ones wake up and they have breakfast until 7:30 - 8:00. I give them toys to keep themselves busy while I make up the beds and clean the rooms. 11:00 I prepare lunch and those from school returns at14: 30; eat and go to rest until 15:30 - 15:45. Then they go to the study room while I start to prepare dinner. I only have a day off in a week of and one weekend per month. I do all the cooking and helping them with their schoolwork… The best reward is the success of the children in your house e.g. when they complete school and get employed. (I get) accommodation, good environment, salary. It 's a very stable situation…. There is no better place for the children. The most difficult thing is to discipline the children,. Last week we had training from (large organisation)on parental guidance and psychosocial support – but we need more training courses, on communication with the children; the children should also be trained on rights and responsibilities… This job is not for anyone, you must love the children against all odds.

I was tested and diagnosed HIV positive in 2001, when I was pregnant with N. I tried abortion, but I was told it was not legalised. So I was trying to get help. My sister somehow met (Director of small organisation) and I joined the support group. That's how I decided to take on this role. Maybe one day someone will volunteer to take care of my child when I die….I was never given pre-test counselling. The post-test counselling was also not really counselling ….I wake up by 5h00. Prepare breakfast. The children go to bed at 8h00. We check on them and change nappies at about 12h00, then at 3h00. After breakfast (usually at 7h00) we clean them. Wash nappies (in machine). Give drugs and vitamins. We then clean the house and dishes. Organise their play. While they play, or watch TV, I prepare lunch. Then feed them or give lunch. We fold clothes. At 15h00 we bath them. 16h00 fruits or yoghurt. 18h00 dinner. Read or talk to them. We rarely have time to read. We just pray with them. We don't get paid as such. Sometimes we get cash. But we are volunteers. We do not expect to be paid. The only thing we get is food and shelter, which we share with the children. We are two full-time staff (for 10 children). We always get a volunteer to release, especially when we are in hospital…Most of (the children in this house)are from poverty stricken families. Mothers are not employed. When we take the children, mothers get the opportunity to go and look for work. We have two orphans. Nobody has so far come up to claim them. ..The ones with parents can go home when parents are stable health-wise, as well as economically. Our problems are the orphans. Maybe if they can be adopted... .. I can't stand it when the kids get sick and you can't do anything for them. It gives me depression. What we need is nutritious food. We find it very difficult to give them all they need, especially those on drugs. (Best thing is that) some of these children had no hope. Many of them, when they came here, you don't believe they will wake up the next day. But now, most of them are well. They are fine. They put a smile on my face. ..Now I think I've got what it takes to live to old age. I want to live my life to the fullest. I am out there doing public speeches, I went public (about my HIV positive status) and I am determined to motivate others.

Stigma and discrimination

Despite existing laws and regulations, children and caregivers in this study were subject to stigma and discrimination in several ways.

Caregivers reported that relatives had deserted/neglected children who were known or suspected to be HIV positive. Some children were 'blamed' for a parental death. In at least one case, a child was barred from kindergarten because his HIV possitive status was known.

> *Everybody was blaming my baby for my sickness. They did not want to touch him because he was positive. They really don't like him and I was thinking of giving him up for adoption.*
>
> Caregiver in rh

> *When I started getting sick and weak my mom suggested that they (father's family) may look after the child for a while but they didn't want to. It hurt me.*
>
> Caregiver in rh

> *Some of their mothers passed away, and their fathers are not interested in them anymore.*
>
> Caregiver in sh

> *We don't tell the other children that he has HIV. But we told the others that when he is bleeding; don't touch it as he has a disease in his blood.*
>
> Caregiver in sh

> *The other boys on the street won't play with S. (because of his HIV+ status)...He goes out anyway and starts kicking the ball...He has taught me so much about courage.*
>
> Caregiver in sh

> *.. some were never visited by any parent or relative. Do you want us to send these children to die of hunger? To be told they are HIV positive and rejected?*
>
> Caregiver in sh

> *I cannot play with other children because my blood is bad.*
>
> Child who is HIV positive

Large organisations and at least one small organisation were active in raising awareness to counter stigma and discrimination:

We advocate. When the need arises I take up issues. We also do radio stations programs. Like now, I am going to UNAM for a call-in program. We try our best to be a mouthpiece for our children.

Caregiver in sh

However there was no evidence in the study region of a centralised plan for a public awareness campaign to counter stigma and discrimination:

A second form of stigma was reported by caregivers in a non-community based setting. They stated that children did not like to be branded as 'orphans'.

They don't want to be told that they are in an orphanage...
When the children complete matric they feel insecure. Because they do not know
what the future looks like. Where they should go.

Caregiver in sh

Effective methods for data gathering

The methodology used to assess services provided to children affected and infected by HIV/AIDS is described above.

A number of processes for data gathering were identified by researchers and research assistants as being particularly useful in the development of this study. It is recommended that these processes be applied to research projects involving sensitive areas such as those associated with HIV/AIDS and care situations for young children.

Firstly, the inclusion of 'voices' of caregivers and children was shown to provide rich data to complement the reports from organisation and centre directors about service provision and outcomes for children. The data was enhanced by use of open-ended questioning and collection of narratives from users of services.

A list of recommended methodological strategies was developed from the study. These strategies were not seen to depend upon large outlays of funds or resources.

The recommended strategies include:

- Identification of a discrete geographical area and target population and identification of major service providers.

- Use of snowball technique to identify smaller service providers and appropriate participants.

- Personal visits by senior researchers to ensure that the goals and parameters of the study are transparent.

- Securing input on interview questions and other data gathering techniques to ensure that participants see value in the study and will benefit from information which is generated.

- Respect for confidentiality at all stages of data gathering.

- Recruitment of research assistants (interviewers) who have similar backgrounds to the re spondents – or similar experiences[17]. RAs should have good interpersonal skills but need not have expertise in the topic of the investigation.

- Provide multi-faceted training to the RAs.

- Provide ways for RAs to interact with respondents in informal and relaxed ways prior to ad dressing interview questions. (This is particularly important when interviewing children). Pre-interview visits are recommended.

- Hold interviews with respondents in their own language and in familiar surroundings to the respondent.

- Make us of audio taping where permission is granted.

- When interviewing children, provide some neutral activity such as colouring or making dough sculptures. This will reduce anxiety and provide a 'talking point' for children.

- Translation of transcripts by research assistants themselves appears to be an effective means of accessing non-English data. (Translations by objective third parties were not trialled).[18]

Lessons from data gathering methods

The collaboration of all persons at every level of service delivery needs to be secured and made clear to respondents. In this study it was deemed that some caregivers may have been unsure about confidentiality and were sensitive about reporting deficiencies in safe houses and elsewhere.

Timelines for data gathering need to be flexible. In this study interviews were often interrupted or rescheduled for a variety of reasons.

DISCUSSION

The varied and different demands and needs for nurturance, stimulation, care, learning, psychosocial and social-emotional support for children at different life stages needs to be taken into account in program development, and delivery and assessment. Survival needs represent just one component

---

[17]. The RAs will have credibility if they have some similar attributes to the respondents such as language, familiarity with the region and/or similar life experience(s). In some cases RAs who represent the target population can be effective in data gathering. However because of confidentiality, it is often advisable to recruit RAs who are not known in the community.

[18]. Comparisons of data when translations are made by an objective third party would be valuable to determine if differences in data presentation occur.

of these needs. It is imperative that any service geared to promoting the wholesome development and well being of children affected and infected by HIV/AIDS should take this into account. (Zimba, Otaala et al, 2002)

Gaps in information

Gaps in current information about the target population were revealed. Data which identifies the number and whereabouts of children, services which are currently being accessed by children and their caregivers and psychological assessments were not available in any comprehensive format. No qualitative or in-depth information about the children which could guide policy and service delivery were found in the public domain. The researchers were unable to uncover previous studies from Namibia which included the 'voices' of children and caregivers.

Without a centralised data base, sustained information gathering and/or vehicles for communication between groups and services will likely remain sporadic, fragmented and/or unequally distributed amongst the target population[19].

There is no evidence of systematic assessment of the quality of current service provision.

Children's needs and rights

It was shown that organisations and services in the study region incorporated many of the attributes of effective early childhood programs and that the full gamut of rights and needs of sample participants were being met in some cases. Many situations, however, did not meet community standards of care.

Needs associated with sustaining health, with access to social and family connections and with cognitive development and school readiness were unmet for many children in the study. Babies in one safe house and children in one residential setting were observed to be living under conditions of questionable hygiene and health practices. Hunger and/or lack of nourishing food were reported by several (residential) caregivers.

Needs associated with psychosocial well-being were deemed to be deficient for the majority of children in this study.

Residential settings

More children from residential settings were reported to be at risk of poor health, poor nourishment or lack of access to school than was reported for other settings.

Many residential caregivers reported feeling exhausted and/or overwhelmed by their role. Nonetheless, children living in residential settings with loving relatives were deemed to have the greatest potential for having rights and needs met. Some factors were shown to qualify the positive attributes

---

[19] CAFO was formed in 2002 as a way to address the need for centralised information and service delivery. They are working towards this goal.

of this situation. Freedom from financial worries and access to programs (such as day programs for preschool aged children, lunch programs and other school support programs for older children) substantially contributed to the health and well being of children and caregivers in this situation.

Most caregivers were in need of support on several levels. Training and support groups could enhance the positive characteristics of this situation. Nearly all caregivers identified a desire to engage in income generation as a way to alleviate financial stresses. Seed grants and consultation on this issue could make a substantial difference to the situation for the children and caregivers.

Safe houses

Children in safe houses generally had their survival needs met, including access to food and shelter and protection from harm. However children in safe houses could be constrained in their psychosocial development and other areas of well-being. A number of factors were seen to contribute to, or constrain, the quality of life in the safe houses. The need for standards of care including space and adult-child ratios, criteria for recruitment and selection of caregivers and appropriate working conditions, were seen to be critical in ensuring that safe houses meet the needs of young children. Infrastructure to supply back-up and emergency care and to ensure accountability and monitoring was similarly shown to be a significant gap in current service delivery.

Children who were isolated by their care situation (in non community-based settings) were branded as orphans causing feelings of exclusion and alienation from community groups. These feelings are likely to be exacerbated as the children mature. Integration into the community wherever possible was seen to be a more sustainable and healthy environment for children.

The majority of caregivers in safe houses in this study did not report feeling overworked or overwhelmed. Caregivers who had a sense of accomplishment and who received support from colleagues and leaders were shown to be motivated, committed and satisfied with their role. Despite illness and poverty in some cases, caregivers in these supportive situations are more likely to provide loving and sustainable care for the children in safe houses than those who were stressed and unsupported in their positions. In one safe house caregivers reported difficult working and living conditions, including having too many children for adequate supervision and lack of privacy for caregivers. Without appropriate standards and supports, the resulting discontent and concomitant turnover in safe houses was likely to have a negative effect on children.

Training

The majority of caregivers were not trained in the provision of experiences for enhancing developmental needs in young children[20]. There is a critical need for training in ways meeting psychosocial needs of young children, in ways of dealing with children experiencing trauma or post traumatic effects and for addressing the special needs of children who are HIV positive. Access to support, personal, specialists and/or consultants to assist caregivers with these issues is highly desirable.

---

[20] One caregiver had training as a preschool teacher. One caregiver was a trained nurse.

Gaps in service provision

While much is being done to address survival and health needs of the target population, needs associated with psychosocial health and well-being were not seen to be adequately addressed in the majority of situations. Meeting these needs depends upon the child's inner resilience, background, ability to make sense of his or her situation and exposure to a health-promoting environment. The caregiver's health and feelings of well-being, consistency in relationships, the availability of 'friends' and the child's success in integrating with others in the neighbourhood and community are further influences of psychosocial health. A description of many of these factors is included in the study. [21]

Services for posttraumatic stress and other therapies were not available to children in this study (many of whom might have benefited from these services).

Programs to facilitate permanent 'family' situation have the greatest likelihood for the long-term health and well-being of young children. A number of organisations mentioned the need for foster families, reunification programs and adoption programs. These types of services are almost impossible for organisations to address without government assistance and/or collaboration involving multiple programs.

Macro system issues: stigma and discrimination

Stigma and discrimination towards children and their caregivers who are HIV positive was found to be widespread. There is a need for public education, awareness raising campaigns and supports to facilitate children in coping with discrimination and self doubts based on their illness, situations and/or status as orphans.

Policy analyses

The parameters of this pilot study did not allow for in-depth analysis of existing and potential policies which affect the target population, including how policies are being implemented under current conditions. A review of relevant legislation and interviews with Ministry officials, including policy decision makers and front line workers, could add important insights into the investigation of service provision. This line of research is recommended for future studies in this area. The *Recommendations Section* below addresses these and other areas which emerged from analyses of the findings.

CONCLUSION

This study gathered qualitative data about the experiences of a sample of children aged 0- 8 years of age who are infected and affected by HIV/AIDS in a designated study region in Namibia (the

---

[21] Empirical assessments of these variable is recommended as a component of program planning and development processes.

target population[22]). The study made use of open-ended questions and observations to provide an insight into what it is like to be young, orphaned, infected or affected in other ways by HIV/AIDS. Situations and settings were described and recommendations made about ways to build on the capacity of current situations in order to ensure the health and well being of the target population.

The study was underlined by the research which describes the influence of the early years upon life-long health and well-being, including the importance of social connections and access to health promoting environments.

The typography of human rights and needs set the framework for investigation. Thus findings focused on the extent to which needs and rights in relation to survival, health and well-being, education and freedom of choice, expression and movement were prevalent in the lives of the target population. The experiences of caregivers and analyses of organisation characteristics associated with quality service provision were included to provide an ecological perspective.

There is little doubt that service providers are aware of deficiencies for children and other members of their communities and are working in many diverse and effective ways to meet these. Organisations, centres and caregivers in the study region are to be commended for the their commitment and selfless provision of services which impact positively upon the target population. In many cases these services are effective in reducing situations which could become critical, even life threatening, for young children.

However the study identified that specific needs of the target population are not systematically documented and not consistently addressed through current service provision.

Two important issues need to be stressed:

The first is that awareness raising about the needs of the 0-8 year old age group is a critical need along with a focus on service development and delivery for this cohort. Perhaps because children who do not attend school are less visible to community groups, it appears that many questions about this population simply remain unasked (e.g. what are their life circumstances and needs?). In this study the inclusion of children's voices assisted in analysing the experiences of this target group. It is recommended that further studies targeting this age group be developed.

The second issue relates to the critical role played by individuals in the delivery of effective services for the target population and others. Community activists, including dedicated staff at all levels and in all settings, appear to be the driving force behind the development and sustainability of service provi-

---

[22] The extent to which the sample is a true representation of all children in the study region was not assessed in any empirical way. However care was taken to ensure that participants represented the three primary care situations for the target population: These were care in residential houses within the community, care in safe houses within the community and care in safe houses which are not community based. Members of the target population who were in residential care and were accessing a daytime preschool program were deemed to constitute a fourth category. Representation from this group was also included in the study.

sion. It is vital that the knowledge base, energy and commitment of these people be acknowledged, rewarded and supported in all ways.

It is anticipated that the findings from this pilot and subsequent studies will be used to raise awareness of the issues, to make recommendations for targeted assistance to the population and to lobby funders and policy makers for further support for research, policy development and for appropriate program support.

Readers are invited to contact the authors for further information about this study[23]

RECOMMENDATIONS

Recommendations are categorised (according to the ecological model) as follows:
Micro system: Recommendations for support to children:

Psychological assessments and information for children and caregivers

Programs

Meso system: Recommendations for Caregiver support:

Training, workshops and support groups for caregivers
Infrastructure and backup
Leadership

Recommendations for organisation support:
Coordination, linkages and support for organisations and service providers.

Exo system: Recommendations regarding policy development and funding issues:
Equity issues
Standards and monitoring
Funding

Macro system: Recommendations for reducing stigma and discrimination.

Recommendations are also included regarding data gathering and research directions.

[23] Jacqueline Hayden, University of Western Sydney; j.hayden@uws.edu.au (see also www.healthychildhood.org)
Cynthy Haihambo, University of Namibia: chaihambo@unam.na
Barnabas Otaala, University of Namibia: botaala@unam.na
Roderick F Zimba, University of Namibia: rzimba@unam.na

Support to children

Psychological assessments, therapies and memory making

There is need to:

1. Develop procedures for assessing the state of health and well-being of OVCs and their caregivers.

2. Make available counselling services, support groups and therapy for post-traumatic stress disorders for children and caregivers who will benefit from these services.

3. Develop record keeping procedures that will ensure children (and caregivers) have informa tion about their backgrounds, including information about their parents and relatives.

Programs

There is need to:

4. Review and enhance services and programs which are specifically targeted at children aged 0-8years of age.

5. Develop and make widely available day programs for young children. These should include an early care and development focus along with the provision of nutritious meals and health services such as health checks and distribution of medicines[24].

   (a) Day programs should include opportunities for providing information and support to caregivers of young children through group meetings, workshops, home visiting and similar programs.

6. Increase programs which support educational and health services to older children includ- ing school lunch and after school tutoring programs, school fee vouchers, school uniforms, and donations of clothes, blankets and other goods.

7. Provide incentives for volunteer programs. Volunteers can be trained and supported to assist with child related activities and provide respite to caregivers. Activities could include excursions, outings, facilitating involvement in sports and other community oriented activities.

---

[24] Accessibility to these types of programs has been shown to alleviate stress for children in residential settings and to address psychosocial and school readiness needs. The programs concomitantly give support and respite to residential caregivers. Availability of these programs will increase the number of children who are able to remain in residential settings. Centre B provides a model for such programs.

Caregiver support

Training, workshops and support groups for caregivers

There is need to:

8.   Provide information about and access to resources for all types of caregivers which address ways to stimulate cognitive, emotional and psychosocial development in young children.

      (a) Facilitate the development of support groups for caregivers.

There is need to:

9.   Provide training and support for caregivers who wish to develop or enhance income genera tion projects.

Infrastructure and backup

There is need to:

10.   Provide a system of 'backup' or emergency care for caregivers in residential settings and safe houses who become ill or are unable to care for the child (ren) in their care for other reasons.

11.   Develop an infrastructure for the recruitment, selection, training and support to caregivers in safe houses.

Leadership

There is need to:

12.   Find ways to develop and reward advocates who take on leadership positions in safe houses and other situations which support young OVCs.

Community and organisation support

There is need to:

13.   Provide incentives for enhanced community involvement to address the needs of OVCs, including those who are infected or affected by HIV/AIDS.

Coordination, linkages and support for organisations and service providers

There is need to:

14.   Provide incentives or other means for allowing time and resources which will facilitate col laboration, networking and linkages amongst organisations, centres, and other service provid ers who target similar populations of children and families.

Policy development and funding issues

Equity issues

There is need to:

15.   Establish a centralized database and to review service delivery which is available to all regions. [25]

Standards and monitoring

There is need to:

16.   Develop a system for identification and monitoring of OVCs, including those aged 0-8 years including information on accessible and needed services for each child.

   (a) Establish a process for updating data on individual children

   (b) Establish a system for collaboration with all relevant agencies to ensure that data is comprehensive and that duplication does not occur.

17.   Develop standards, monitoring processes and code of conduct for caregivers in safe houses.

   There is need to:

   (a) Establish standards for working hours, duties and salaries[26].

   (b) Monitor the number of children and age/sex combinations to ensure healthy relation ships can be established in the home.[27]

Funding

There is need to:

18.   Investigate current funding policies from the Ministry and to monitor current use of this funding source[28].

---

[25] This will assist in ensuring that children and families have equal access to services, regardless of geographical location.

[26]Efforts to alleviate heavy workloads and financial concerns will allow for more time to be spent taking care of the caregiver herself and in positive interactions with children. This should reduce turnover of staff and concomitant disruption and distress for children.

[27] Some young children are disadvantaged by being in a house with many older children whose needs take precedence.

[28] The N$10 per day allowance was reported to be too restrictive and may be inadequate to cover children's needs. This could be encouraging caregivers to take in larger numbers of children, which decreased the quality of life for the children and caregiver. There is a need for accountability and/or standards in service delivery which can be tied to this funding.

19. Review criteria and assess procedures for support to organisations and caregivers from the Ministry and other donors;
    (a) Investigate the potential for increased support from government sources and other agencies for identified needs of the target population.

20. Coordinate funding and other support from Ministries and other reliable, long-term sources as a means to increase access to existing sources, reduce duplication of funding and identify targets for new or redirected funds.

21. Investigate the potential for accessing corporate sponsorship;

    (a) Provide assistance to organisations to learn about diverse fund raising techniques.

Sustaining existing programs and developing new programs

There is need to:

22. Develop an infrastructure (collaborative network amongst policy decision makers and service providers) which will allow for consistent assessment of service delivery and of changing needs, and

    (a) Make use of the infrastructure to plan and develop new programs as needs emerge.

23. Provide seed grants and/or other supports to facilitate the development and implementation of sustainable income generation projects for caregivers.

24. Enhance and develop new programs aimed at recruiting foster families, reunifying families and relatives with children and, where appropriate, adoption of children.

Reducing stigma and discrimination

There is need is:
25. Provide incentives for programs of public education and awareness raising aimed at de creasing discrimination for children and adults who are HIV+.

26. Review and ensure compliance with anti discrimination laws and policies for children and adults who are known to be HIV+.

27. Find ways to further integrate children in non-community based settings to counter branding as orphans, and other sources of stigma.

Data gathering and research directions

There is need to:
28. Assess the situation of young OVCs and their caregivers through studies which include

qualitative data, as well as quantitative measures, including descriptions of the experiences of caregivers and narratives which incorporate children's perspectives.

29.   Develop a process whereby data concerning the target group are updated on a regular basis.

REFERENCES

Barry, F. (1996). Endangered children and environmental standards. *Community Development, 4*(2), 3-6.

Carnegie Corporation of New York. (2000). *Mobilize communities to support young children and their families.* Retrieved 22/06, 2000, from http://www/carnegie.org/starting_points/startpt5.html

Clarke, S. H., & Campbell, F. A. (1989). Can intervention early prevent crime later? The abecedarian project compared with other programs. *Early Childhood Research Quarterly, 13*(2), 319-343.

Cox, E. (1995). *A truly civil society.* Sydney: Australian Broadcasting Corporation.

Dahlberg, G., Moss, P., & Pence, A. (1999). *Beyond quality in early childhood education and care: Postmodern perspectives.* London: Falmer Press.

Doherty-Derkowski, G. (1995). *Quality matters: Excellence in early childhood programs.* Ontario: Addison Wesley.

Ferguson, D. M., Horwood, J., & Lynskey, M. T. (1994). A longitudinal study of early childhood education and subsequent academic achievement. *Australian Psychology, 29*(2), 110-115.

Gahan, C., & Hannibal, M. (1999). *Doing qualitative research using QSR NUD*IST.* London: Sage Publications.

Hayden, J. (2002). Early childhood developments in Zimbabwe: A community centred approach to extraordinary circumstances. In L. Chang & E. Mellor (Eds.), *International Developments in Early Childhood.* (pp. 239-251). New York: Peter Lang.

Hayden, J., & Macdonald, J., J. (2001). Community centred childcare: A new answer to 'who benefits'? *Australian Research in Early Childhood Education, 8*(1), 33-40.

Hayden, J., & Macdonald, J. J. (2000). Health promotion: A new leadership role for early childhood professionals. *Australian Journal of Early Childhood Education, 25*(1), 32-38.

Hiner, C. (2000). *Working with NUD*IST: A plain English guide to using QSR NUD*IST 4.* Mtubatuba, South Africa: The African Centre for Population Studies and Reproductive Health.

Kandetu, V. (2000). *Review and Update of Resources for Vulnerable Children in Namibia.* Windhoek: Ministry of Health and Social Services and UNICEF.

Kawachi, I., Kennedy, B. P., & Glass, R. (1999). Social capital and self-rated health: A contextual analysis. *American Journal of Public Health, 89*(8), 1187-1193.

Leeder, S. (1998). Social capital and its relevance to health and family policy. *Australian and New Zealand Journal of Public Health*(August), 3-12.

Lero, D. S. (2000). Early childhood education - An empowering force for the 21st century? In J. Hayden (Ed.), *Landscapes in early childhood education: Cross national perspectives on empowerment.* (pp. 375-385). New York: Peter Lang Publishers.

Love, J. M., Schochet, P. Z., & Meckstroth, A. L. (1996). *Are they in any real danger? What research does and doesn't tell us about child care quality and children's well being.* Princeton, NJ: Mathematical Policy Research, Inc.

Lust, D. & O'Gara, C. (2002). The two who survive: the impact of HIV/AIDS on young children, their families and communities. HIV/AIDS and Early Childhood. *Coordinators' Notebook: An international resource for early childhood development pp3-21.* No. 26. The Consultancy Group on Early Childhood Care and Development.

Lust, D.; Huffman, S.L.; and O'Gara, C. (2000). *Assessment and Improvement of Care for AIDS-Affected Children Under 5.* Washington, D.C.: International Centre and Care and Education for Children.

Marmot, M., & Wilkinson, R. G. (Eds.). (1999). *Social determinants of health.* Oxford: Oxford University Press.

Maslow, A. H. (1970). *Motivation and personality* (2nd ed.). New York: Harper.

Maton, K. (2000). Making a difference: The social ecology of social transformation. *American Journal of Community Psychology., 28,* 25-57.

McBride, S. L. (1999). Family centred practices: Research in review. *Young Children, 54*(3), 62-70.

McCain, M., & Mustard, J. F. (1999). *Early years study. Reversing the real brain drain. Final report.* Toronto: Ontario Children's Secretariat.

Ministry of Health and Social Services (MHSS) (2001). *Orphans and Vulnerable Children Five-year Strategic Plan for 2001 - 2006 and Programme Proposals for 2002 - 2003.* Windhoek, MHSS

Moss, P. (1995). *Defining objectives in early childhood services.* Paper presented at the European Conference on Quality of Early Childhood Education, Paris.

Nicholson, J., Tually, K., & Vimpani, G. (2000). Establishing research priorities in early childhood health inequalities. An overview of the Australian research contribution and identification of priority areas for research. Paper presented at the Health Inequalities Research Collaboration Child, Youth and Family Research Network, University of Newcastle.

Parcel, T. L., & Menaghan, E. G. (1994). Early parental work, family social capital and early childhood outcomes. *Social Psychology Quarterly, 99*(4), PP 972-1009.

Pence, A. R. (1999). It takes a village and new roads to get there. In D. P. Keeting & C. Heertzman (Eds.), *Developmental Health and the Wealth of Nations: Social, Biological and Educational Dynamics.* London: Falmer Press.

Qualitative Solutions and Research Pty Ltd. (1997). *QSR NUD*IST* (2nd ed.). La Trobe University, Victoria: Qualitative Solutions and Research Pty Ltd.

Schweinhart, L., & Weikart, D. (1993). Success by empowerment: The high scope perry preschool study through age 2-7. *Young Children, 49*(1), 54-58.

Shonkoff, J. P., & Phillips, D. A. (2000). *From neurons to neighbourhoods: The science of early childhood development.* Washington DC: Office of Educational Research and Improvement.

Steinitz, L. (1998). *Resources for Vulnerable Children.* Windhoek: Ministry of Health and Social Services, and UNICEF.

Steinitz, L. (2002). Oral presentation made at a UNESCO/UNAIDS sub-regional workshop on "Combating HIV/AIDS through education: The case of street children in Southern Africa",

Harmony Seminar Centre, Windhoek, Namibia, 15 - 19 April, 2002.

Subbaro, K.; Mattimore, A.; and Plangemann (2001). *Social Protection of Africa's Orphans and Other Vulnerable Children: Issues and Good Practice Program Options*. Washington, D.C.: Human Development Sector, Africa Region, the World Bank.

Summary of the National Children's Forum on HIV/AIDS held in South Africa, (2001) (author)

The Children's Institute. (2001). *The national children's forum on HIV/AIDS preliminary report. "Children can make a change – hear our voices!"* Retrieved 16 June, 2004, from http://www.pmg.org.za/docs/2001/appendices/010928Forum.htm

UNICEF. (1994). *Children and women in Zimbabwe: A situational analysis update*. Harare: UNICEF.

United Nations General Assembly. (1948). *Universal declaration of human rights*. Retrieved June 16, 2004, from http://www.un.org/Overview/rights.html

United Nations General Assembly. (1989). *Convention on the rights of the child*. Retrieved May 22, 2000, from http://www.hrweb.org/legal/child.html

United Nations International Children's Fund. (2002). *The state of the world's children*. Retrieved June 16, 2004, from http://www.unicef.org/sowc02/pdf/sowc2002-eng-full.pdf

USAID, UNAIDS, & UNICEF. (2002). *Joint report details escalating global orphans crisis due to AIDS: Number of children orphaned by AIDS will rise dramatically. Press release, Barcelona, 10 July 2002*. Retrieved June 16, 2004, from http://www.usaid.gov/press/releases/2002/pr020710.html

Vinson, T. (1999). *Unequal in Life: The distribution of social disadvantage in Victoria and NSW*. Richmond: Ingnatious Centre for Social Policy and Research.

Wadsworth, M. (1999). Early life. In M. Marmot & R. G. Wilkson (Eds.), *Social determinants of health* (pp. 44-57). Oxford: Oxford University Press.

Wilkinson, K. (2000). The cold hand of rationalism that depletes community spirit. *Rattler*(54), 26.

Wong, R. S. K. (1998). Multidimensional influences of family environment in education: The case of socialist Czechoslovakia. *Sociology of Education, 71*(1), PP 1-22.

Wong, S., & Patterson, C. (2000, January). *Teachers' theory of multicultural education*. Paper presented at the Australian Research in Early Childhood Education Conference, Canberra, Australia.

World Bank. (2000). *Investing in our children's future. Case studies. Background papers for session IV, how can the private sector influence public policy*. Washington DC: World Bank.

Zigler, E. F., & Gilman, E. D. (1998). Day care and early childhood settings: Fostering mental health in young children. *The Child Psychiatrist in the Community, 3*, 483-498.

Zimba, R. and Otaala B (2002). *An Assessment of Services for Young Orphans, Older Orphans and other Children Affected and Infected by HIV/AIDS in the Caprivi, Erongo, Karas, Kavango, Khomas, Ohangwena, Omaheke and Oshana Regions Of Namibia*. Proposal submitted to Ministry of Women's Affairs and Child Welfare, Government of Namibia.

APPENDIX I

INTERVIEW QUESTIONS

1.1   Interview Questions for Representatives from large and small Organisations

1. What services do you provide for OVCs (and/or children who have been infected/affected by HIV/AIDS)?

2. Do you have any special services for children aged 0-8years?

3. Can you explain how the services are able to be provided (funding? donation? etc)

4. Is your funding secure? Do you think your organization will be functioning 2-5 years from now?

5. Can you estimate the number of children aged 0-8 years who are receiving some services from you?

6, Do you have any way of knowing if all OVCs (0-8 years of age) in your catchment area have access to your services?

    6.1 Can you estimate what percentage of OVCs of this age group are known about and/or accessing services?)

    6.2 How do the children/caregivers access your services?

7. How did this service(s) come to be developed?

8. Can you prioritise the services which you think are needed for this age group in your catchment area?

9. To what extent are you able to meet (or coordinate others to meet) these priority needs within your organisation?

10. How else might (could) these priority needs be met?

11. Can you recommend services to children/families in this age group which would prevent some of the needs from developing?

12. What or who is the driving force behind the programs?
    Would you say that they fit into one or more of these categories?

- Community driven – developed and adopted by community needs

- Community based – takes place in the community where most recipients live

- Community operated – are run by people in the community?

13. Do you think that your programs which include services for children aged 0-8 are 'holis tic' that is do they attempt to cover all needs (health, nutrition, education, psychosocial and practical support such as reunifications, income generation, and others…)

14. Do your programs raise awareness of the needs of children infected and affected by HIV/AIDS? How do they do this?

15. Do your programs have direct links with other programs such as schools, health services, nutrition etc? If so how are these developed and maintained? If not, why not?

16. Do your programs have a system for human resource sustainability and perpetuation – that is, is there training, apprenticeships or other ways that new workers can come into the system?

1.2 Interview Questions for Care Givers

Introduction

We would like your home to be part of a study about what services are available for OVC – especially for children infected and affected by HIV/AIDS who are below the age of 9 years. The information from this study will be sent to agencies and organisation and may facilitate the development of policies and supports for these children.

The interview will be audio recorded and then transcribed. Your name will not be used in the final report – nor will the home be identified– so you should feel free to give any information to us. It will remain confidential. You should feel free NOT to answer any question if you do not want to.

Only myself – the research will hear the tape. I will record your answers and then destroy the tape. No one other than myself will know who said what in this study.

Your home was recommended by____.
If you agree to this study can we have the following information from you?

About the setting

1. Please name the children in this house and their ages (first names only)
2. Do you know how many of the children are infected?
3. Can you tell us a little bit about the children in the house under 9 years?
   i. Why they are here…
   ii. How long have they been here for?

    iii. Is there somewhere else they could go?

    iv. What will happen to them in the next 2 years?

4. How many people take care of the children?

5. Can you explain the roles and responsibilities of caregivers n this setting

    i. What hours do they work

    ii. Do they have time off?

    iii. Do they receive any kind of support or pay? (If yes, from whom? How much?)

About the caregiver

6. *Can you tell us how you came to take on this role of caregiver for these children?*

7. Can you tell us about your own 'story' or situation?

8. Do you get support or help from any source in this role?

9. What kind of support or help would you like?

10. What do your daily responsibilities as caretaker entail? (Can you describe what you do on a typical day?

11. What has been your most successful or memorable experience in caring for these children?

12. Can you tell us some other good things that have happened here?

About the children

13. What do you see as the most important needs of these children? Please list up to 4 needs.

14. How are these needs being met now?

15. Which needs are not being met now?

16. How could the needs be met (what would you need or who else could be involved to make sure that the needs are met?)

17. What kinds of things do the children in your care do every day? (Do they have a chance to play or do other activities – what do they like doing the best?

18. To summaries – what are the 3 best and the 3 hardest things for the children here?

    1. What are the 3 best and the 3 hardest things for you working here?

Thank you for your help with our study.

I.3 Interview Questions for Children

Introduction

Here are paper and markers. Please draw a picture of about your home here?

What do you want me to write about this picture?

NOTE: Tell the child "I will leave the materials so that you can draw as many pictures as you like later. Would you mind talking to me for a few minutes – there are things I would like to know. You can continue to draw while we talk if you like."

A very young child (or one unfamiliar with paper and markers) can use dough instead of pictures: ask them to make a model of anything – e.g. a person – ask 'who is that – what can you tell me about this person'? etc

If children are too shy to draw they can be asked to tell a story – the interviewer can draw a picture for them about their story.

---

1. How did you come here?
2. Who takes care of you (gives you food, clothes, helps you when you feel sick?
3. Do you have brothers, sisters or any other relatives here with you?
4. Do you have friends here now?
5. Who is your best friend – or person you like the most in the world? Are they here with you? Do you ever see them?
6. What is good about being here (what do you like the best?)
7. What would you like to change about being here?
8. What do you want to become when you grow up?
9. Is there anything you would like to tell me about living here?

Observations

1. Child's level of communication skills (ability to respond, initiates communication, seems able to express feelings).
2. Child's general demeanor (eye contact, smiles, talkative, friendly, withdrawn, tearful)
3. Child's perceived level of health and wellness (including cleanliness, nutrition, etc)
4. Other comments.

APPENDIX II

RESEARCH PROPOSAL ORIGINALLY SUMBITTED (2002)[29]

FOR FUNDING

AN ASSESSMENT OF SERVICES FOR YOUNG ORPHANS, OLDER ORPHANS AND OTHER CHILDREN AFFECTED AND INFECTED BY HIV/AIDS IN THE CAPRIVI, ERONGO, KARAS, KAVANGO, KHOMAS, OHANGWENA, OMAHEKE AND OSHANA REGIONS OF NAMIBIA

Proposed Research Team
Researchers
Research Assistants

Proposed Advisory Inter-sectoral Committee
A representative from the Ministry of Women Affairs and Child Welfare
A representative from the Ministry of Basic Education, Sport and Culture
A representative from the Ministry of Health and social Services
Two representatives from the University of Namibia
A representative from UNAIDS, Windhoek office
A representative from UNICEF, Windhoek office
A representative from UNESCO, Windhoek office

A representative from the Association of Early Childhood Care and Development

A representative from Catholic AIDS Action
A representative from the Legal Assistance Centre
A representative from the National Orphans and other Vulnerable Children
(OVC) Steering Committee
August, 2002

---

[29] Persons/Organisations interested in supporting this project should please contact:
- Professor Rodericik F. Zimba, University of Namibia, Private Bag 13301, Windhoek, Namibia
Telephone: 264 61 206 3647; Fax: 264 61 206 3980; Email: rzimba@unam.na Or
- Professor Barnabas Otaala, University of Namibia, Private Bag 13301, Windhoek, Namibia
Telephone: 264 61 206 3312; Fax: 264 61 206 3320; Email: botaala@unam.na

Background

Recently, UNESCO and UNAIDS commissioned situational analyses of HIV/AIDS among children in difficult circumstances in Lesotho, Namibia, Swaziland and Zambia (Chisepo, 2001; Haihambo-Muetudhana, Zimba and Nuuyoma-Kalomo, 2002; Maphalala, 2001; Mwaba and Mbewe, 2001). These analyses yielded four reports that represented a serious effort at enhancing our understanding of the impact of adversity on children in difficult circumstances (CDCs) in the four countries. How the HIV/AIDS pandemic exacerbated and perversely implicated every aspect of the children's social-cultural, social-economic and psychosocial deprivation, exploitation and hardship was amply captured in the four reports. Furthermore, governmental and non-governmental efforts and actions to ameliorate the adverse effects of the rather squalid conditions and circumstances under which the children were made to exist were informatively communicated in the reports.

While describing the services supplied to CDCs, the reports provided rich information on constraints the four countries faced when doing this. For instance, all the four country reports referred to a lack of adequate resources to confront the daunting problems of large numbers of HIV/AIDS orphans, street children, child sex workers, children with special needs, working children and other vulnerable children who required medical and educational services and needed to have their basic needs for shelter, food, security, protection from disease and other forms of harm met.

The other constraints referred to were the following:

> It was reported, in some of the countries, that the provision of services to CDCs was done in the context of a policy vacuum. This robbed service providers of health, educational, legal and other guidelines of how to cater for the children. Related to this was the absence, in all the four countries, of performance indicators that could be used to assess the impact and quality of services provided to CDCs. This placed many service providers in a situation where they were unable to evaluate the quality of the impact of their work.

> Most service providers for CDCs did not have specific and clear programmes on HIV/AIDS issues affecting the children. These providers placed more focus on survival issues confronting these children. Moreover, no clear information on how zero to 8 years of age children affected and infected by HIV/AIDS were catered for was provided in the reports.

> Several programmes for CDCs placed little emphasis on the developmental, social-emotional, psychosocial, nurturance and other well-being aspects affecting these children. This was taken to be unfortunate as what CDCs needed most was psychosocial support, nurturance and care. They badly needed healing from trauma and on-going struggles for not only physical but also psychological growth and development. This was not being adequately provided in some of the four countries.

> The severe strain on the extended African family was given as another serious constraint that hindered the provision of effective services to CDCs. As an important source of **social-cultural and psychosocial resilience** and **healing,** this traditional African resource was no

longer available in the form it used to be in the four countries. Deaths through HIV/AIDS had weakened and disrupted this **reservoir of resilience** even further. I addition to strengthening the extended family system, **transformed, restructured and reconstructed community support mechanisms** and **belief systems** needed to be put in place and formalised.

There appeared to be no mechanism for assessing and monitoring the quality of services provided to CDCs. This called for more comprehensive periodic situation analyses on these services. Such analyses should use indicators for assessing the quality of services offered to the CDCs (Zimba, 2002).

A number of these constraints were confirmed at a UNESCO/UNAIDS sub-regional workshop on "Combating HIV/AIDS through education: The case of street children in Southern Africa" that took place at Harmony Seminar Centre, Windhoek, Namibia during the period of 15-19 April, 2002. Officially opened by Namibia's Minister of Women Affairs and Child Welfare, the Honourable Netumbo Ndaitwa and attended by representatives from Botswana, Lesotho, Malawi, Namibia, Swaziland, Zambia and Zimbabwe, the workshop provided very little information on **specific services provided to street children aged 3-8 years who might be affected and infected by HIV/AIDS.** Due to this, the quality of such services could not be ascertained for all the countries represented at the workshop.

Notwithstanding the concerted efforts that are being taken to mitigate the impact of HIV/AIDS in the health, social, educational and other sectors, the paucity of information on the quality of **differentiated** services provided to young children aged 0-8 years and older children aged 9-18 years who are affected and infected by HIV/AIDS prevails in Namibia. In the educational sector for example, very little is known about how early childhood development and education programmes in the country infuse in their operations concerns regarding young children affected and infected by HIV/AIDS. What has in fact been observed in a recent study on the impact of HIV/AIDS on education in Namibia is the need to lay HIV/AIDS prevention foundations during the early years of life, to appropriately nurture, care for, support and socialise young children affected and infected by HIV/AIDS in pre-schools and other caregiving contexts (Abt Associates South Africa Inc., 2002).

The information made available at the *First National Conference on Orphans and other Vulnerable Children* in Namibia does not provide evidence about how well these and other young children affected and infected by HIV/AIDS are cared for (Government of the Republic of Namibia (GRN), UNICEF, Family Health International (FHI) and USAID, 2001). **Aggregated** and **differentiated** information on how well the young and the older children were catered for by several service providers was also unavailable at the *Second National Orphans and other Vulnerable Children Conference : Facing Challenges, Ensuring Futures* that was held on 25-27 June, 2002 at Safari Hotel in Windhoek, Namibia (GRN, UNICEF, FHI and USAID (2002). Services for children aged 0-8 years and those aged 9-18 years who are affected and infected by HIV/AIDS seem not to have been **delineated** and **differentiated according to their specific developmental needs and rights.** The latest situation analysis of orphan children in Namibia does not also clarify matters on this aspect. What it does is merely describe some adjustment emotional problems some of these children experience. It does not provide information on the quality of development-related services that the young children are provided with (SIAPAC, 2002). This gap in understanding and knowledge needs to be filled up with research information.

It should be recognised though that a comprehensive directory of resources for Namibian vulnerable children was prepared in 1998 and reviewed in 2000 (Steinitz, 1998; Kandetu, 2000). The resources annotated in the directory are provided by government ministries and NGOs. In addition, it should be noted that NGOs such as the Catholic AIDS Action and the AIDS unit of the Legal Assistance Centre provide services to young children affected by HIV/AIDS and their families. For instance, the Catholic AIDS Action provides caring and other services to 9 885 orphans and vulnerable children who are members of 1 625 family units through out Namibia (Steinitz, 2002). A cadre of volunteers is trained by the NGO to provide home-based family care (Futter, 2000). However, the point to note is that no information on the quality of resources available to vulnerable children has been located. Moreover, it is not clear from the information available, which specific resources are for young children affected by HIV/AIDS and which are not. Furthermore, plans that have been put in place to mitigate the impact of HIV/AIDS by the Ministry of Basic Education, Sport and Culture do not include the issue of monitoring and evaluating the quality of services provided to young children affected by HIV/AIDS (Ministry of Basic Education, Sport and Culture, 2001). Inconsistent with this, a Five-Year (2001-2006) strategic plan for orphans and vulnerable children and its programme proposals covering 2002-2003 that has been prepared by the Ministry of Health and Social Services does include the aspect of monitoring and evaluating the quality of services for the children (Ministry of Health and Social Services, 2001). However, **no** monitoring and evaluation information on services for young orphans and other children aged 0-8 years and children aged 9-18 years who are affected and infected by HIV/AIDS is provided. What is available is a plan to gather this information.

As was indicated earlier, the lack of focus on monitoring and evaluating services that cater for young and older children affected and infected by HIV/AIDS is not unique to Namibia. In *Children Orphaned by AIDS: Front-line responses from Eastern and Southern Africa* (UNAIDS and UNICEF, 1999), a variety of services offered to Tswana, Malawian, Zambian and Zimbabwean children affected by HIV/AIDS are described. Little information is provided in the document on how the quality of the services is monitored and evaluated.

The justification for the study

The importance of paying attention to the quality of services that young and older children affected and infected by HIV/AIDS receive and ought to receive could be communicated by the following reasons:

> Monitoring and evaluating the services would direct the focus of support to young and older children's developmental and age-appropriate needs. As is well known, infants, toddlers, children aged 3-6 years, 7-9 years, 10-12 years and those aged 13-18 years have varied and different demands and needs for nurturance, stimulation, care, learning, psychosocial and social-emotional support. Survival needs represent just one component of these needs. It is imperative that any service geared to promoting the wholesome development and well being of children affected

and infected by HIV/AIDS should take this into account. In their seminal study on the ***Assessment and improvement of care for AIDS-affected children under age 5,*** Lust, Huffman and O'Gara (2000) give empirical evidence and policy justification guidelines for this position. Furthermore, Ainsworth and Semali (2000) support the position by providing empirical evidence on the adverse impact of HIV/AIDS on the health and development of the affected children. They demonstrate how incidences of morbidity, stunting, nutritional wasting, and failure to thrive can attend these children. The negative effects of these characteristics on intellectual development and performance have been well documented over the years.

The Convention on Children's Rights demands that all children should be protected from various forms of harm, abuse, neglect, exploitation and deprivation. It demands that all children have an inherent right to life, optimal development and to an enriching standard of living (UNICEF, 1989). Children affected and infected by HIV/AIDS are entitled to all these rights. There is evidence to the effect that some services for these children can expose them to abuse, neglect and exploitation. For instance, foster care can be given in such a way that it involves "stigmatisation and discrimination in food allocation, education and workload" (Subbarao, Mattimore and Plangemann, 2001, p.24). Deininger, Garcia and Subbarao (2001) express a similar sentiment when they state that the costs to children affected and infected by HIV/AIDS could include "the strong possibility of dropping out of school, a decline in nutritional status, possible increase in child labour, — discrimination and exploitation". Ainsworth (1992), found that foster children engaged in more labour intensive economic activities than foster parents' own children. In addition, she found out that foster children had less access to education than foster parents' own children. Monitoring and evaluating services for children affected and infected by HIV/AIDS would reduce instances of the violation of their rights.

Monitoring and evaluating services for young and older children affected and infected by HIV/AIDS would ensure that early childhood development issues and well-being, cognitive and psychosocial developmental matters implicating older children are considered and taken into account by service providers, including communities, educational systems, NGOs and donor agencies. There is a tendency to downplay these issues when articulating global strategies for mitigating the impact of HIV/AIDS on key sectors such as that of education. For instance, the World Bank has given scanty attention to early childhood and psychosocial matters in its latest book on **Education and HIV/AIDS: A window of hope** (The International Bank for Reconstruction and Development/The World Bank, 2002).

Evaluation results of services offered to children affected and infected by HIV/AIDS could form the basis for improving and enhancing these services. For instance, the findings from the study could be used by the line government ministries of Women Affairs and child Welfare, Basic Education, Sport and Culture and Health and Social Services to strengthen services and review policies for young orphans, older orphans and other vulnerable children affected and infected by HIV/AIDS. Furthermore, the findings could enable other service providers for the children to ***reorient*** and ***refocus*** their services with the aim of making them more **developmentally differentiated, adequate and appropriate.** Households and communities could also be supported and strengthened when caring for their orphans and other vulnerable children affected and infected by HIV/AIDS.

The research task

Based on the preceding background, the task in the proposed study will be to assess services Namibia provides to young orphans, older orphans and other children affected and infected by HIV/AIDS with the intention of strengthening programmes and communities offering the services. Young children affected and infected by HIV/AIDS referred to here are those aged 0-8 years and older children affected and infected by HIV/AIDS are those aged 9-18 years. Moreover, services in question will include those of a cognitive and psychosocial development nature, health and nutrition, education and social-economic ones. In the area of education, emphasis will be on the degree of access children aged 7-18 years have to schools and the extent to which they are enabled to remain in school. In addition, programmes in operation and those envisaged for the benefit of these children will be looked at. Moreover, we shall explore the impact of teacher attrition due to HIV/AIDS on the quality of education these and other children receive.

Objectives of the study

The objectives of the study will be to:

1. identify programmes that provide services to young orphans aged 0-8 years, older orphans aged 9-18 and other children infected and affected by HIV/AIDS;

2. delineate the nature of services that are provided to the young orphans, older orphans and other children affected and infected by HIV/AIDS;

3. ascertain whether the services provided relate to the developmental, psychosocial and other well-being needs of young orphans, older orphans and other children affected and infected by HIV/AIDS;

4. find out whether the services provided to young orphans, older orphans and other children affected and infected by HIV/AIDS take into account the rights of the children, especially the rights that pertain to protection from abuse, neglect, exploitation, stigmatisation and discrimination;

5. identify specific cognitive development, psychosocial development, child care and development constraints and strengths pertaining to orphans and other children affected and infected by HIV/AIDS that households, communities, governmental and non governmental service providers have;

6. generate information to be used in the review of the overall National policy on children and propose policy and programme strategies for serving Namibian children affected and infected by HIV/AIDS more adequately.

Methodology

Population

Although we have no definite statistics on households in Namibia with children affected and infected by HIV/AIDS, we can reasonably assume from data provided by Catholic AIDS Action that there are thousands of households with these children all over the country. The exact number of children affected and infected by HIV/AIDS served by governmental and non- governmental organisations is unavailable.

For our purposes, the population of our study will be all representatives of households with young orphans, older orphans and other children affected and infected by HIV/AIDS in the specified regions of Namibia. Moreover, we shall also include, in the population, all governmental and non-governmental service providers.

Sample

Using systematic stratified sampling, 10% of the households with children affected and infected by HIV/AIDS will be drawn from the selected 8 Namibian political regions. More accurate estimates of the number of households to be reached by doing this will be specified after consultations with stakeholders.

Because of financial and other constraints it is prudent to gather data from 8 regions of the country only. It should be noted that all selected regions have been ravaged by the HIV/AIDS pandemic. In fact, the impact of the pandemic has been more horrific and devastating in the majority of the selected regions than in other regions. Representatives of all known governmental and non-governmental service providers will also be included in the sample.

It is hoped that the remaining 5 regions of the country will be covered in the second stage of the study.

Research measures

To assess the households' capacity for providing young orphans, older orphans and other young children affected and infected by HIV/AIDS with optimal protection, health care, early childhood care and development, access to primary and secondary school education, nutrition, housing, cognitive/psychosocial stimulation and family/community support, a number of research measures will be employed. These are:

•	an adapted household survey instrument prepared by the *Task Force for Child Survival and Development* (World Bank, Early child Development Team, 2001) will be employed;

•	adapted research materials developed by the *International Centre on Care and Education of young children;*

•	an instrument containing interview questions for older orphans and other older children affected and infected by HIV/AIDS will be developed;

- focused group discussion questions for key service-provider informants will also be developed.

Procedure

A number of steps will be taken to conduct the study. These are:

1. A multi-sectoral *advisory* committee consisting of governmental, NGOs, UNAIDS, UNICEF, UNESCO and the University of Namibia members will be constituted.
2. With the support of the advisory committee, a research team consisting of researchers and research assistants will be formed.

3. Using ECD, ECCD, psychosocial and social-cultural theoretical perspectives, a more comprehensive integrated literature review to clarify the research task and to further guide the research process will be prepared.

4. Once adapted, the research instruments and the interview questions will be translated from English into local languages spoken in the 8 regions. To ensure that the translated questions remain conceptually the same, other independent translators will translate them back into English.

5. Research instruments will be pre-tested

6. Researchers and research assistants will hold a training workshop on the conduct of the project prior to the commencement of data collection.

7. Logistical preparations before visiting regions to collect data will be made.

8. In the regions, research instruments will be administered to household principal caregivers of young orphans, to older orphans, to other older children affected and infected by HIV/AIDS and to other information rich persons by trained research assistants. Researchers will supervise these assistants. In appreciation of their services, household respondents will be given an honorarium. Moreover, research assistants will conduct focused group interviews with representatives of communities, governmental and non- governmental service providers.

Data analysis

Frequencies, cross-tabulations and other descriptive statistics will be used to analyse most of the quantitative data. Frequency tables and figures will be used to present the data. Qualitative interview data will be coded, categorised and synthesised to generate meaningful themes and recurring patterns from it.

Draft budget*

Item	Approximate cost in US Dollars
Transport/travel	11 000
Researches', research assistants' and field research costs	25 000
Production and translation of research materials, stationery, adn procurement of literature review material	11 500
Research assistant training and local dissemination workshops	11 200
Regional workshops	8 000
Telecommunication and postage	700
Data coding, entry, analysis and report writing	6 000
Payment of token of appreciation to respondents	7 000
5% contingency for inflation	4 020
TOTAL	**84 420**

* This is a **draft** budget. It is open to revision.

REFERENCES

1. Abt Associates South Africa Inc.(2002). *Draft Summary Report on the Impacts of HIV/AIDS on Education in Namibia.* Paper submitted for discussion by education sector stakeholders at a dissemination and planning workshop that took place on 26-27 March, 2002, Safari Hotel Conference Centre, Windhoek, Namibia.
2. Ainsworth, M. (1992). *Economic Aspects of Child Fostering in Cote d'Ivoire.* Washington D. C. : World Bank.
3. Ainsworth, M. and Semali, I. (2000). *The impact of adult deaths on children's health in North Western Tanzania.* Washington D. C. : World Bank.
4. Chisepo, L. (2001). *Situation analysis on HIV/AIDS among children in difficult circumstances in Lesotho.* Maseru: Department of Social Welfare, Lesotho.
5. Deininger, K., Garcia, M. and Subbarao, K. (2001). *AIDS-induced orphanhood as a systematic shock: Magnitude, Impact and Program Intervention in Africa.* Washington D. C. : World Bank.
6. Futter, M. (2000). *Home based family care in Namibia: A practical manual for trained volunteers.* Windhoek: Catholic AIDS Action.

7. Government of the Republic of Namibia (GRN), UNICEF, FHI, USAID (2001). *First National Conference on Orphans and Other Vulnerable Children: Summary Report.* Windhoek: GRN, UNICEF, FHI, & USAID.

8. GRN, UNICEF, FHI, USAID (2002). *Second National Orphans and other Vulnerable Children Conference: Facing Challenges, ensuring Futures,* June 25-27, Safari Hotel Conference Centre, Windhoek, Namibia. Unpublished conference proceedings.

9. Haihambo-Muetudhana, C. K., Zimba, R. F. and Nuuyoma-Kalomo, E. N. (2002). *National situation analysis on HIV/AIDS among children in difficult circumstances in Namibia.* Unpublished research report.

10. Kandetu, V. (2000). *Review and update of Resources for Vulnerable Children in Namibia.* Windhoek: Ministry of Health and Social Services and UNICEF.

11. Lust, D., Huffman, S. L. and O'Gara, C. (2000). *Assessment and improvement of care for AIDS-affected children under 5.* Washington D. C. : International Centre on Care and Education for Children.

12. Maphalala, T. (2001). *A situation analysis of HIV/AIDS among children in difficult circumstances in Swaziland.* Kwaluseni: University of Swaziland.

13. Ministry of Basic Education, Sport and Culture (MBESC) (2001). *Strategic and operational planning for the management and mitigation of HIV/AIDS in the Namibian Education Sector.* Windhoek: MBESC.

14. Ministry of Health and Social Services (MHSS) (2001). *Orphans and vulnerable children five-year strategic plan for 2001-2006 and programme proposals for 2002-2003.* Windhoek: MHSS.

15. Mwaba, R. and Mbewe, M. (2001). *National situational analysis on HIV/AIDS among children in difficult circumstances in Zambia.* Lusaka: Zambia National Commission for UNESCO.

16. Steinitz, L. (1998). *Resources for vulnerable children.* Windhoek: Ministry of Health and Social Services and UNICEF.

17. Social Impact Assessment and Policy Analysis Corporation (SIAPAC), Ministry of Health and Social Services (MOHSS) and UNICEF/Namibia (2002). *A Situational Analysis of Orphan Children in Namibia.* Windhoek: SIAPAC, MOHSS and UNICEF.

18. Subbarao, K., Mattimore, A. and Plangemann, K. (2001). *Social protection of Africa's orphans and other vulnerable children: Issues and good practice program options.* Washington D. C.: Human Development Sector, Africa Region, the World Bank.

19. UNAIDS and UNICEF (1999). *Children orphaned by AIDS: front-line responses from eastern and southern Africa.* New York: UNAIDS and UNICEF.

20. UNICEF (1989). *The convention of children's rights.* New York: UNICEF.

21. World Bank (2002). *Education and HIV/AIDS: A window of Hope.* Washington D. C.: The World Bank.

22. World Bank (2001). *Child Needs Assessment Tool Kit: A tool kit for collecting information your organisation needs for designing programs to help young children in areas heavily impacted by the HIV/AIDS epidemic.* Washington D. C.: World Bank, Early child development team.

23. Zimba, R. F. (2002). *Preface to reports on situational analyses of HIV/AIDS among children in difficult circumstances in Lesotho, Namibia, Swaziland and Zambia.* Windhoek: Namibian Commission for UNESCO.